CAREERS IN
COSMETOLOGY

By
ELIZABETH STEWART LYTLE

The Rosen Publishing Group, Inc.
NEW YORK

Published in 1999 by The Rosen Publishing Group, Inc.
29 East 21st Street, New York, NY 10010

Cover photo by Ira Fox

First Edition

Library of Congress Cataloging-in-Publication Data

Lytle, Elizabeth Stewart.
    Careers in cosmetology / by Elizabeth Stewart Lytle. — 1st ed.
      p. cm. — (Careers)
    Includes bibliographical references and index.
    Summary: Describes some of the different careers in cosmetology, the training and education required, licensing requirements, future job possibilities, and more.
    ISBN 0-8239-2889-6
    1. Beauty culture—Vocational guidance—Juvenile literature.
[1. Beauty culture—Vocational guidance. 2. Vocational guidance.]
I. Title. II. Series: Careers (Rosen Publishing Group)
TT958.L97   1999
646.7'2'023—dc21   99-11568
                                 CIP

Manufactured in the United States of America

About the Author

Elizabeth Stewart Lytle is a photojournalist, teacher, and communications consultant in western Pennsylvania. This is her fourth book in the Rosen Publishing Group's career series. Other titles by the author are *Careers in the Construction Trades, Careers for Electricians,* and *Careers in Plumbing, Heating and Cooling.*

A former state director of the Pennsylvania Women's Press Association, Mrs. Lytle has received several writing awards as a newspaper journalist and as a freelance magazine writer. She was also nominated, in 1991, by the Franklin Area School District for the Sallie Mae First-Year Teacher Award, a program recognizing 100 of the nation's most outstanding new educators.

She and her husband are the parents of one son.

Acknowledgments

This book would not have been possible without the support and encouragement of many people and organizations interested in the field of cosmetology. The author wishes to acknowledge Daryl Hicks, owner of the Classic Salon, Oil City, PA, for sharing his expertise; Jayne Morehouse and Norma Lee, public relations contacts for the Cosmetology Advancement Foundation; the National Hairdressers and Cosmetologists Association; Milady and Salon Ovations Publications, and the many professional cosmetologists who contributed time and information.

Dedication

For Rowan McGuire Lytle, who arrived June 12, 1997, and has taught me to view the world with wonder again; and for Christian and Erin K. McGuire Lytle.

Contents

1

Help Keep America Beautiful—
Become a Cosmetologist

Imagine getting to do creative work in glamorous surroundings. Now think of what it would be like to start a career after only one year of training. And wouldn't it be great to finish that training and find that you have many different job opportunities to choose from? This is a reality for thousands of professional cosmetologists. Professional cosmetologists work in settings that vary from neighborhood beauty shops to elegant salons and spas. Every day more than two million Americans visit cosmetologists seeking professional advice and services to help them look their best.

A cosmetologist is trained to perform an array of care and treatment services that enhance personal grooming and appearance. In addition to helping their clients look good, skilled cosmetologists provide a psychological boost as well.

THE BASICS OF COSMETOLOGY
Cosmetologists provide cosmetic services, products, treatment, and advice. In addition to shampooing, cutting, and styling hair, they may also color, curl, or straighten it by a chemical process. An array of care and treatment services related to the skin and nails are also within cosmetologists' duties. Their training may cover

topics such as massage and electrolysis (the removal of unwanted hair). It is important that cosmetologists understand both chemistry and anatomy, as these sciences relate to their work.

Cosmetologists in neighborhood beauty shops are called generalists. This means they practice many or all of the various aspects of their training. They may provide hairstyling, manicuring, skin care, and other related beauty services. Those employed in large salons may specialize in only one or two areas of service. Cosmetologists who work at spas are usually specialists. They may center their training on therapeutic massage, aromatherapy, or giving facial treatments. Some cosmetologists specialize in mixing and applying hair color—a part of the hair-care industry that is growing rapidly—or the related specialty involving wigs and hair extensions. These are created, styled, colored, and cared for by specially trained technicians. Technicians who specialize in skin care are called estheticians.

Today's salons may also include indoor tanning facilities and manicure booths, as well as exercise facilities and cosmetic counters. The "day of beauty" approach, where clients spend the better part of an entire day being pampered and groomed, is gaining popularity in many salons.

Cosmetologists can work in a variety of locations and have many different job titles. Those who specialize in selecting cosmetics that will enhance a client's appearance are in demand from small towns and big cities to Hollywood movie studios. In urban areas, experienced cosmetologists often work as image consultants and might actually represent manufacturers of beauty products. They may also work as platform artists, displaying products and illustrating techniques at trade shows. Photo stylists and fashion consultants are also in demand.

Within a well-run salon, cosmetologists operate as creative designers, working closely with people on the cutting edge of fashion. Many of these professionals also enjoy a comfortable income.

The cosmetology industry also offers opportunities for those who are interested in business. You could become the owner-operator of your own salon, or you could manage a chain of salons. If teaching appeals to you, why not consider becoming a cosmetology instructor?

WIDE-OPEN FIELD

Success in the field of cosmetology has few limits. Currently, quality beauty services are in high demand. A recent national study of the salon business indicates that opportunity exists for thousands of additional employees, but there are simply not enough stylists trained to fill these positions.

While many professions require college degrees and years of experience, more than half the openings in the beauty industry are for entry-level jobs. In many states, a cosmetologist can gain the skills for this career in one year of full-time practice and theory classes. Deserving students who lack financial resources have many opportunities for financial aid. If you are in the early years of high school, you may be eligible for free technical education, leading to a high school diploma and the chance to take the cosmetology licensing exam in your state.

IS THIS A CAREER FOR YOU?

Cosmetology is a popular career choice, offering many rewards and challenges. Most people who work in the beauty industry are enthusiastic about their career. They are rewarded daily by seeing the results of their time and talent. They also get feedback from satisfied clients.

There are many naturals in this field—people who are drawn to the world of design and fashion by some instinct or talent. Often these people are impeccably groomed and sport the latest hairstyle or fashion accessories. This is the person your friends turn to for a quick French braid after gym class. In the library, a future cosmetologist may be found poring over the latest fashion magazines. At the movies, this person's focus maybe be studying the actors' clothes and hairstyles, rather than focusing on the plot.

In the pages that follow, you will meet successful cosmetologists as well as students who are preparing for their future careers. Through their words and ideas, you will gain a clear view of what it is like to earn a living in the beauty industry. This book attempts to look at a career in cosmetology from all angles, the pros and cons, rewards and challenges. Our goal is to help you make an informed and important decision about your future.

2

The Beauty Industry Through the Ages

Humans have long been interested in improving personal appearance. Grooming techniques and ornamental adornments have been part of human society since long before written records were kept. Archaeologists exploring the sites of civilizations dating back to 4000 BC have unearthed ancient cosmetic containers and toiletries.

Ancient peoples of Egypt, Sumaria, Israel, and Babylon left records of an interest in cosmetic practices. An early form of eye shadow known as kohl was found at many dig sites. Drawings of people from that era often show the use of dramatically outlined eyes or eyebrows, created through the application of this dark-colored substance.

Excavation of an Egyptian pyramid yielded an ornate cosmetic box packed with gold-rimmed jars of cosmetics, silver rouge dishes, mirrors, and a razor. The Egyptians were especially taken with adornment of the hair and eyes. At one time in Egyptian history, noblewomen shaved their heads and wore stylized wigs in brilliant hues of blue, red, green, or glossy black. Scented oils and colorings were used to groom the hair. The Egyptians were even known to experiment with various treatments to combat baldness.

Eye makeup was likewise dramatic. The area beneath the eyes was frequently painted green, using powdered malachite. Egyptians also used cosmetics to disguise facial wrinkles. They would apply a compound of oil, wax, incense, and ground cypress berries to the skin. Cleopatra was known to mix honey into her famous milk baths as a part of her beauty regime. Honey is a humectant, or substance that keeps the skin's natural moisture from evaporating, and is an ingredient commonly found in facial creams even today.

The ancient ceremonial art form of body painting called Mehndi began in India and is used in many cultures. Mehndi is a temporary design applied to the skin surface using an artist's brush and a paste made from a safe organic substance called henna. Henna has long been used as a reddening agent for temporary hair coloring.

Ancient people of the Mediterranean region used perfumes and false hair, along with eye makeup for both men and women. The Greeks amassed great knowledge of herbs and plants with which they concocted dyes for their hair and pigments to add color to their cheeks and lips. The elite of Scythia slathered their entire bodies in a paste made of frankincense and ground cedar and cypress woods mixed with water. After a full day of this treatment, the paste was gently washed away, resulting in skin that was smooth and glossy.

At first, the Romans showed more interest in constructing roads and building a huge empire than in improving their own appearance, although they did approve of the use of hot mineral baths for therapeutic value. After conquering the Greeks and Egyptians, however, Roman citizens, both male and female, adopted some of those civilizations' cosmetic practices. Hair bleaches, lip and cheek rouge, eye makeup, powders for the face and body, perfumes, and hair oils all became popular with fashionable Romans. They invented dressing rooms and had slaves to assist them in dressing and grooming procedures. Many women had a female slave called the ornatrix, whose primary role was to skillfully apply cosmetics and create ornate hairstyles.

The fall of the Roman Empire sent the use of cosmetics into decline throughout much of the world. Only the Arabs maintained an interest in cosmetic arts during this period of history. Perfumes, powders, and eye makeup were used by women of the desert cultures. In Europe, there is little mention of cosmetics until soldiers and pilgrims began returning from the Crusades with cosmetics acquired in their eastern journeys.

The Renaissance in Europe brought a revival of interest in makeup and personal adornment, and scientific advances brought a new level of sophistication to their manufacture. Both men and women in aristocratic circles used powders for the face, body, and hair. Perfumes and toilet waters were distilled, and hairstyles took an elaborate turn. It was said that Queen Anne of England used a blend of honey and oil to keep her long hair thick and lustrous. Among the poor, beet juice was used to tint lips and cheeks, while flour meant for baking was diverted for use as face and body powder.

HISTORY OF HAIR

To achieve long-lasting curls and waves, women in early Egyptian and Roman civilizations were known to apply a mixture of soil and water to their hair, wrap it on wooden rollers, then bake it in the sun. Of course,

7

the results were messy by our standards, and certainly not permanent.

According to hair historians at the Vidal Sassoon headquarters in Europe, during the sixth century in Rome only prostitutes were blonde. Eventually bleaching processes overcame this societal stigma, and anyone who desired a change and who could afford the process felt free to lighten his or her hair color.

In the mid-1400s aristocrats took to shaving their eyebrows and along the hairline of their foreheads in order to mimic the profiles of classical sculpture. Three centuries later, big hair was in, for men and women alike. The theory was that the bigger your hair, the higher your station in life.

By the mid-1600s, a very vain King Louis XIV of France and his court were setting fashion trends for the world to follow. Members of Louis XIV's court at Versailles began the fashion of wearing wigs. The look was particularly popular with men, who chose shoulder-length styles with tightly rolled curls falling in rows. Fashioned of human hair, they were heavy and designed with flaps over the ears and at the nape of the neck, to make it easier to turn one's head. They were expensive to buy and to maintain. Because they needed to be washed, dried, and styled, most people owned at least two wigs, and many owned several different styles. In one shape or another, wigs remained the essential accessory of the upper classes for over a century. Wigs even had a place in the courtrooms of England well into this century.

In the late 1870s, hair extensions had become common, often in the form of spiral curls attached at the crown. Then, in 1900, Charles Dana Gibson, a *Life* magazine illustrator, created a drawing of a young woman with a loose, messy hairdo. The Gibson Girl style became the rage. To achieve the look, many women acquired the new permanent wave, which could take up to twelve hours to process.

In 1905, Charles Nessler invented a perming process that was effective but depended on electrical current for its use. Women sat beneath a heavy, rounded device similar to a salon hood-type dryer, while curling rods wired to the device were wound into the hair. The beauty operator had to be careful not to let the rods actually touch the scalp, for fear of electrocuting the client.

By the 1920s, many American women were cutting their long hair. This bobbed style led to the invention of the croquignole (KROH-ki-nol) wrapping technique, which yielded deep waves with loose curls at the ends. The first chemical-action perms were invented by chemists in 1932.

Less than a decade later, another method of permanent waving was introduced. First a lotion was applied, to soften and expand the hair strand. After this waving lotion had done its chemical work, another lotion called a neutralizer was applied to harden and shrink the hair strand, enabling it to conform to the shape of a curling rod around which small sections of hair were wrapped. This process was called a "cold wave," since it did not depend on heated rollers. The alkaline perm, still popular today, is a modern version of these early cold waves.

Over the next two decades, motion pictures began to affect popular culture and fashion. By 1931, short bobs and the platinum blonde look became popular with movie stars. Achieved through the use of harsh bleaches, however, platinum was a look that caused a lot of damage to many women's hair.

High fashion in the mid-1950s became defined by the beehive hairdo, achieved with vigorous back-combing and hairspray. By 1959, London was becoming a trend-setting city for the next new look in hair and fashion. This Mod style was the definitive look of 1960s British youth culture. Clothing designer Mary Quant introduced the mini skirt, while hairstylist Vidal Sassoon introduced the shaped haircut, launching an influence in hair design that would leave its mark for the next four decades.

By the mid-1960s, fashion had begun to swing back to more conservative styles. High school yearbooks across the United States showed evidence of a hairstyle called The Flip, basically a smooth pageboy with the ends flipped up. Not just a style for the young, versions of it were worn by women from ages fifteen to fifty.

In the 1970s, hairstyles tended toward the free-flowing and romantic, which came to a rather abrupt end a decade later with the punk look, another import from London. Of course, hairstyles vary in their ability to attract devotees, and few women were tempted by the next craze, a brief flirtation with "bald is beautiful," which struck in the mid-1980s. By 1988, slick hairdos and pompadours created with gel, mousse, and hairspray reached a peak of popularity.

For the '90s, there is no one dominant look. Any length or texture is appropriate, so long as the hair itself is in top condition. We are entering an era of extreme freedom in hair history. Consumers are expressing more interest in natural, botanical hair-care products and geometric cuts that provide movement. Hair coloring is now a highly refined science that treats hair as an important accessory and provides sophisticated methods for highlighting or contrasting individual skin tones.

THE HISTORY OF NAILS

Smooth hands with nails that were long and colored were considered a sign of high social status among ancient peoples. The gilding of nails, with gemstones attached, was a common practice among the leisure class. To remove unwanted cuticles, people rubbed them with sand. Sharp stones served as nail files. Only the men received manicures in ancient Greece, and those were performed by barbers.

Nail colorings were derived from henna, the same Asian shrub used for hair coloring. Women in ancient Turkey boiled rose petals to make a pink coloring for their nails. Another method evolved in China, where people used a nail color derived from chicken blood.

Manicures and nail treatments have come a long way since then. At one time, only nobility indulged in manicures and pedicures, but today such treatments are thought of as an integral part of good grooming. Although for some time now, men have sported clear nail polish to top off a manicure, in general, colored nail polishes have been used exclusively by women. The latest marketing coup is nail polish for men, in colors with names such as Sand, Mica, and Concrete.

THE RISE OF AROMATHERAPY AND MASSAGE

The ancient Greeks were among the first to explore what is today called aromatherapy, the use of botanical perfumes to enhance well-being. They believed that perfumes had a mythological origin.

From a scientific standpoint, aromatherapy is the use of pure essential oils, extracted from many parts of plants. These may include not only flowers and leaves, but also resin, bark, roots, twigs, seeds, berries, rinds, and rhizome. Products made from these botanicals are used to relax and rejuvenate the body, mind, and spirit.

Sometimes considered a form of folk medicine, aromatherapy is mentioned in the histories of both Egypt and India more than 4,000 years ago. Egyptians created massage oils, medicines, embalming preparations, skin care products, fragrant perfumes, and cosmetics from aromatic plants. Similar materials were used in India as part of the ancient medical practice known as Ayurveda.

Doctors and scholars in England and France were part of a movement in the early 1900s that prompted a revival of the benefits of natural medicine and aromatherapy, with a more recent revival dating to the early 1990s. Today in England and the United States, aromatherapy is a commonly accepted alternative medicine. In France, it is even more widely accepted, with pharmacies selling essential oils and some health insurance companies reimbursing for such treatments.

Considered both an art and a science, aromatherapy is not yet an exact science. There is general agreement about the actions of certain oils, but textbooks vary in their descriptions of the properties and characteristics of an essential oil. The exact effect of its use often varies among individuals.

Massage has been known for centuries, but its practice in the United States is relatively new, dating to the early 1900s. Massage stimulates the body's soft tissue—muscles, skin, tendons, and ligaments. The touch used can be light or heavy. The masseuse employs various techniques to stroke, tap, brush, gently hold, or rub the flesh. The results are muscle relaxation, relief of stress and fatigue, and stimulated circulation of blood and lymph. Massage is intended to increase health and well-being.

Trade shows in the beauty industry now devote attention to such spa topics as aromatherapy and massage treatment. A type of Oriental massage technique called Shiatsu is currently popular.

Whole-body massage, also known as Swedish massage, is the technique associated with health clubs and physical therapy. Eastern methods such as acupressure, based on identified pressure points, and reflexology—which emphasizes a connection between pressure to certain areas of the foot and the well-being of various internal organs and functions—are often used as well. Estheticians use gentle facial massage to improve blood circulation and muscle tone.

As a cosmetologist, you will be able to add your own unique methods to the ever-changing history of fashion. You will contribute to the evolution of techniques for promoting health and beauty and be part of the great influence of style on popular culture.

3

Career Possibilities

Cosmetology jobs are found in various settings, from small-town business districts to malls, department stores, cruise ship salons, and movie sets. The average starting salary in 1998 varied from $12,000 to $16,000, moving up to $25,000 after five years in the business, and to about $32,000 after ten to fifteen years.

Cosmetology is one of the fastest-growing careers in the nation. Last year, four job openings were available for every new cosmetologist who had earned a license. Each year, more men and women turn to professionals in the beauty industry for increasingly specialized services. The demand for pampering services such as pedicures and massage is growing. These procedures help clients deal with the stress of their daily lives.

By the year 2000, this country will need an additional 82,000 professionally licensed cosmetologists. You could be one of them.

WHAT COSMETOLOGISTS DO

According to the National Cosmetology Association in St. Louis, Missouri, a licensed cosmetologist is qualified to do manicuring, shampooing, permanent waving, hairdressing, facial and scalp treatments, haircutting, hair coloring, eyebrow shaping, skin care, body care, makeup, and chemical hair treatments. Here are job titles associated with the beauty industry today: Manicurist; Nail Technician; Hairdresser; Wig Technician; Image Consultant; Color Specialist; Permanent Wave Technician; Natural Hairdresser; Skin Care Specialist/Esthetician; Cosmetic Artist; Retail Specialist in Beauty Products; Specialist in Aromatherapy and Massage; Theatrical Makeup Artist; Platform Artist; Cosmetology School Instructor; Salon Manager; Salon Owner; and Freelance Cosmetologist.

Hairstyling has become a very technical field. Such issues as the shape of the client's face, skin tone, and natural hair color and texture must all be considered in achieving a cut that is flattering and also meets the client's needs in terms of facilitating upkeep.

Hairstyles are created through a variety of methods, usually dictated by the client. The cosmetologist may curl or add body to the hair by giving a permanent wave or, conversely, straighten curly hair by means of a chemical hair-relaxing process. Hair bleaching and coloring treatments are also commonly performed, as are scalp treatments.

Among services increasingly in demand are those that make the hair seem fuller or longer by means of weaving in artificial extensions. Such hairstyles are complex and time-consuming to achieve, requiring that the extensions be secured to the client's own hair. The look known as a million braids is one example of a style created with hair extensions. As you might imagine, styles using extensions are considerably more expensive than more traditional styles, yet they can also last for several weeks with only minor touch-ups.

A cosmetologist is also trained to give facials, shape and tint eyebrows and eyelashes, do makeup analysis, and demonstrate various products and techniques, plus style and care for wigs and hair extensions. Some individuals give their clients facials and/or neck massages.

There are salons in which cosmetologists specialize in one or more aspects of beauty services. Someone who has taken only the short course in manicuring must limit his or her work to services related to nail care. A manicurist cleans, shapes, files, and polishes nails and cares for the cuticles. Applying and caring for artificial nails is another skill common among manicurists. Because nail art has become so popular, some particularly creative and talented manicurists have specialized in creating nail art, hand-painted with an air brush in detailed, multi-hued designs or created with decals. Nail technicians are also well versed in artificial nail technique and maintenance, including linen and silk wraps.

Some salons include electrolysis service, the permanent removal of hair from skin. There may also be esthetic treatments to cleanse and beautify the skin. General cosmetology training covers both subjects, but usually these are areas in which a cosmetologist may specialize.

As the spa industry continues to grow, the need for individuals trained in massage therapy increases. The client may sit in a specially designed massage chair or lie on a table while the massage is performed. The client remains fully clothed during a chair massage, whereas other types of massage have the client covered with a towel or sheet for warmth and modesty.

A cosmetologist is licensed to perform services similar to barber-stylists, except that a cosmetologist cannot shave facial hair. At one time, barbers were restricted to male clients, but times have changed, and with that change came the onset of the unisex salon.

CONTINUING EDUCATION

On top of working scheduled hours, salon owners and managers hold regular staff meetings when the shop is closed, using this time to discuss matters related to business operations, or to bring employees up to date on the latest techniques or products.

Many salons provide continuing educational opportunities for their staff, either through part-time enrollment in beauty academies or by underwriting the cost of seminars and professional workshops. Knowledge acquired in these ways is often shared with coworkers during staff meetings. Experts in the professional beauty industry recommend that operators take part in a five-day refresher course each year. The time can be divided between a spring styling show and annual state conventions held in the fall.

Other continuing education opportunities for hairdressers are sponsored by manufacturers of hair-care products, particularly perms and hair colors. Sessions on cosmetic science and hair analysis are also available, presented at the firms' headquarters or at a beauty academy.

MANAGERS AND OWNERS

The salon manager checks supplies and equipment, makes appointments, handles accounts, does bookkeeping, purchases all merchandise, and sees that all legal regulations are met. There are a limited number of manager's jobs, however, since the salon owner is often the manager and may also serve clients.

The largest financial return comes from owning the salon, but there are also risks and responsibilities tied to this position. An individual needs capital to invest, thorough training in the cosmetic arts, and business ability to make a salon succeed. In the early days of launching one's own business, the salon owner may do all the work, adding additional staff as the volume of business builds.

Salon owners are responsible for operating expenses and payroll. How much time they devote to serving clients varies. Some simply greet clients when they arrive and spend the rest of their time running the business or supervising the staff. Other owners continue to operate a work station. Stylists are paid 40 percent to 50 percent of the gross sales they bring in. After meeting expenses, the owner is free to call the difference profit.

Increasingly, the modern salon depends on profits from retail sales of hair-care and beauty products. Some salon owners have a real talent for marketing, offering such products as rain capes, hats, and umbrellas in the spring; gift certificates for salon services as Mother's Day or prom/graduation gifts, sunless tanning products in the summer, and stocking-stuffer grooming aids during the holiday season.

Savvy business operators use specialized computer programs to forecast when a client will need a new perm or color service. They may also actively market a certain product with the use of phone calls or written reminders. The accent is on personal service, but the technique builds business volume for the salon.

A NON-LICENSED OPTION
There is one job in a beauty salon that does not require a cosmetologist's license, and that is the position of receptionist. This is the first person a client sees

and talks to, so it is important that receptionists demonstrate a friendly and caring attitude as soon as people walk through the door. It makes good business sense to hire a receptionist who is outgoing, attentive, and, hopefully, good at putting names and faces together correctly.

A receptionist has many duties to perform. Clients arrive and must have their appointments confirmed politely and promptly. The phone rings all day with requests for appointments, changes, cancellations, calls for the staff, and various requests to be routed. Receptionists announce the arrival of clients to the cosmetologist with whom they are booked and may even be called upon to help supervise small children who accompany their parents on salon visits.

As a receptionist, you can expect to recommend services and products that the salon offers. This will require advanced knowledge on your part, and some attention to the basics of salesmanship. Additionally, at the start or end of your day, you may be expected to help clean the shop or restock merchandise.

Through it all, you will be keeping the book in which appointments are recorded for the entire staff. More and more hair salons now use computerized records, so you may need to have some computer skills. Some receptionists take responsibility for tracking details of the services a client obtains on each salon visit. A print-out of their last visit may be produced and given to the stylist when the client returns.

While a salon receptionist does not need a cosmetology license to perform these duties, many who start out behind the desk make the decision to go to cosmetology school after observing the career in action.

OPPORTUNITIES OUTSIDE THE SALON

Today's cosmetologists are not just those you see in salons, shops, and spas. Remember that the people on stage or behind the scenes at a beauty show, or even in front of a cosmetology school classroom, represent career choices that may be available to you.

There are several career options within this field. For instance, platform artists are experienced, creative cosmetologists who spend all or part of their time demonstrating the newest looks and introducing new beauty products during industry trade shows. These usually occur in civic centers or auditoriums, where thousands of participants, all professionals in the beauty industry, register to attend. It is also possible that a platform artist would visit a large salon, particularly one associated with leading manufacturers or large chains, and make a presentation for the staff.

Those with an advanced certificate in cosmetology, plus practical experience, may work as a cosmetology instructor. There are hundreds of schools in which to work, from vocational high schools to community colleges and privately owned career centers. Instructors in cosmetology schools need additional hours of training, plus a second licensing exam to move up from the salon.

Those with specialized talents may become beauty magazine writers or editors, image consultants, or theatrical makeup/hair stylists, working backstage in live theater or for film companies. Others work as examiners for state licensing boards or become sales representatives for cosmetic firms.

IF SHOW BUSINESS BECKONS

Is there much demand for hairdressers to the stars? You can judge for yourself by reading the credits of movies and TV shows that you watch. Just a casual glance at the close of a recent action-adventure movie revealed that each of the leading actors had his or her own hairdresser on the set. A popular soap opera routinely lists the names of four hairdressers who work behind the scenes.

Many cities have production companies and photographic studios where commercials and advertisement materials are created. There are other similar opportunities for makeup artists to work in their hometowns, which will be discussed later. But first, let's explore the world of the professional makeup artist.

After acquiring their basic training, these professionals may specialize in the costume and hairstyles of various historic eras, learn how to use cosmetics to age a character over a lifespan or create special-effects makeup to mimic burns or wounds.

There are four basic categories of makeup specialties. Live work is the term used to describe makeup for day, evening, or glamorous occasions. There is another category for still photography, under natural or artificial lighting. An example of this would be makeup for models featured in advertisements. The two additional specialty areas are makeup for actors in stage productions and and makeup for film actors.

Surprisingly, not all the jobs in this field are in Hollywood. For example, a directory of makeup artists in Arizona lists professionals who do hair, makeup, and special effects for print work, commercials, film, fashion, sports, and industrial filmmaking. Even in the desert communities of Phoenix, Scottsdale, and Tucson there are professionals who work on films that range from Disney productions to *Star Trek* and the Academy Awards live broadcasts.

Even if you never live in Hollywood or work with stars of the highest magnitude, you may discover a creative outlet in your own hometown, providing makeup and hairstyling for school plays, community theater productions, dance recitals, or ballet, opera performances, and special events.

Whether your adventures as a makeup artist take you backstage just a few times a year or become the foundation of your cosmetology career, you are sure to enjoy the exciting world of show business. To learn more about careers in this field, contact the International Alliance of Theatrical Stage Employees, the labor union joined by most professional makeup artists.

EARNINGS

What a cosmetologist earns depends on the size and location of the salon, patrons' tipping habits, competition in the area, and the ability of a hairstylist to attract and hold regular patrons. As is the case with many jobs, a certain amount of "paying your dues" that with new and relatively inexperienced workers. But practice makes perfect, and after investing some time and hard work, stylists and nail techs can develop a following of their own, make better wages, and gather larger tips.

Typical entry-level pay for large chains is $12,000 annually, plus customer tips. At present there is no clear-cut information on the amount by which tips boost a cosmetologist's earnings, but it is reasonable to expect 10 to 15 percent of the cost of service.

According to the *Princeton Review Guide to Careers*, starting salaries were up to $15,000 industry-wide, moving up to $24,000 after five years and $31,000 with ten to fifteen years of experience. Top pay for a stylist is about $45,000 annually, according to the beauty industry's *Green Book* report.

Much of the increase in cosmetology pay in recent years reflects the impact of supply and demand. Increased emphasis on the sale of beauty products has also increased earning power. Remember, too, that a cosmetologist receives tips, generally 10 to 15 percent of the service fee, from most clients. In the beauty industry, there are several basic methods for calculating employee compensation. They are:

Straight Salary

This is usually paid to a salon manager who performs client services only when all other operators are busy. The manager's regular duties include bookkeeping, making bank deposits, ordering supplies, etc. A manager who regularly performs client services generally earns the same percentage as beauty operators, in addition to his or her straight salary.

Straight Percentage

Straight percentage is typically 50 to 60 percent of the business an operator is directly responsible for in a week. A senior designer—an operator with extensive training and experience—may earn a higher percentage. Commissions on merchandise sales are usually treated separately.

Dual Percentage

Dual percentage is a method similar to straight percentage except that services performed are priced individually. For instance, shampoos, hair treatments, and rinses are paid at a standard rate, but tints, bleaches, toners, scalp treatments, and so on are paid at a lower rate, to cover the cost of supplies. General work may be paid at a rate of 45 percent, but special work would pay only 40 percent of gross.

Operator-Purchased Supplies
Operator-purchased supplies are a method by which the beauty operator pays for supplies used (for example, a permanent wave kit) and the percentage wage is figured at a standard rate.

Sliding Percentage
In this method, after reaching a specified gross sales figure, the percentage rises for the next block of sales. Generally sales blocks are in increments of $100. For example, a cosmetologist earns 40 percent on the first $100 in gross sales; 45 percent for the second $100, 50 percent for the next, and so on.

Profit Sharing
In this method, all operators, regardless of the number of hours they have worked, earn the same percentage on their gross salary. After salon earnings reach a predetermined figure, a certain amount of profit goes to the employees. The percentage is figured according to an operator's gross total during the period. The sum is added to the operator's paycheck as a reward for working hard. This system encourages cooperation among the staff, since the total that coworkers bring in may increase your earnings.

Booth Rental Agreements
In a booth rental agreement, the salon owner rents a work station to a beauty operator, with or without supplies. The owner pays a larger percentage to the operator, since the

stylist is now self-employed, freeing the salon owner from the responsibility of paying taxes and insurance on the stylist. This method is not legal in all states. Check for the laws in your state before agreeing to this type of arrangement.

Combination Plans

Combination plans are mix-and-match arrangements reflecting elements of any method listed above, so long as the salary structure is mutually agreeable to salon owner and staff.

The salary schedule is something you have a right to discuss during a job interview. If the prospective employer does not raise the subject voluntarily, you can tactfully ask which method of compensation the business uses. Of course, you will learn more about this aspect of the career during your formal training.

Figures from the professional beauty industry indicate that a salon invests more than $3,000 in hiring a new graduate. This figure covers the cost of advertising, special sales promotions, and of course, the salary guarantee.

Industry-wide, there is an inexperienced worker in one of every four salons. However, two out of every five working cosmetologists have been at the same salon for three or more years.

FRINGE BENEFITS

Large salons and department stores now generally offer group life and health insurance, as well as other benefit plans. These benefits are also available in smaller shops, but the employee may have to work at the location from six months to a year in order to qualify. Nearly all employers provide annual paid vacations of at least one week after a year of service.

Some cosmetologists, both employees and salon owners, are members of the United Food and Commercial Workers International Union. Professional makeup artists have their own union, associated with the film industry.

GETTING AHEAD

Advancement for the cosmetologist usually comes in the form of higher wages as you gain experience and build a steady clientele. Some salons pay advancement bonuses as stylists gain more experience and advance from a junior to a senior level.

Another method for advancement is to relocate to a center of fashion and the performing arts. New York and Los Angeles have long been recognized as such centers. Pittsburgh, Miami, Toronto, and Vancouver are emerging as popular movie locations used by major production companies. These cities offer many opportunities for cosmetologists to become hairstylists and makeup artists to the stars. You can learn more about professional makeup artists in chapter 5. Jobs are also available as makeup artists and hairstylists for on-camera performers in even the smallest TV broadcasting stations. The same is true for metropolitan theater and opera companies.

A SALON OF YOUR OWN

Another route is to become the manager of a single shop or a chain of salons. About half of all cosmetologists become business owners by acquiring the necessary license to open their own salon. This may be a privately held business or a franchise operation.

In most states, there are two routes by which cosmetologists acquire the combination of training and experience required to pass the salon management licensing exam. The first method requires that the individual with a state cosmetologist's license complete additional hours of training in a state-certified school or academy before taking the management exam. The second method requires that applicants work full time in a licensed shop for a period of time, often two years, before sitting for the same written exam. Much like an apprenticeship, the work experience should expose the would-be salon manager to the business aspects of running the shop. Study guides are also available to help them prepare for the exam.

Most owners are based in a salon location, but increasingly, freelance cosmetologists take their services to the client. Either way, a good cosmetology program includes step-by-step business training. The industry offers other short courses and informative books that will help you plan and establish your business venture. If you are motivated, you will surely find the right program to prepare you to open and manage a salon of your own. You will learn how to finance the venture, equip your salon, hire and manage a staff, operate on a budget, and grow your business.

4

Is This a Career for You?

There are currently 630,000 people working in the cosmetology profession; 90 percent of them are women. A
high proportion are self-employed salon owners. This
indicates that cosmetology is a great place for the entre-
preneur. Most cosmetologists work forty hours a week,
including evenings and Saturdays. Busy times during
the year include holidays, graduation, and the wedding
season. During these times many cosmetologists work
four to eight hours overtime per week.

Just as cosmetology offers abundant opportunity for
those who want to devote long hours to their career, it
is also a field that can provide a part-time or flexible
schedule. A significant number of cosmetologists work
part time, citing flexible hours as one of the most
attractive features of this career.

TRAINING

Compared to many jobs, cosmetology training is short,
hands-on, and quite specific. You learn to perform a
variety of personal care services, to communicate effectively with clients, to handle various chemical processes,
learn how to run a business, all in about one year of full-
time classes.

Thousands of courses are available in a variety of
educational settings ranging from vocational-technical

high schools to career academies and community colleges. If you are in your mid-teens when you decide to become a cosmetologist, you can obtain your training at little or no cost through vocational high school programs. Other students find financial aid available through grants and loans, or enroll in a part-time program that allows them to work while they learn.

Since the fifty states set their own rules about how much training a cosmetologist must have, the standard varies from state to state. For example, California requires 1,600 hours of instruction, while Florida requires 1,200 hours; Kansas and New York require 1,000 hours each, and Pennsylvania, 1,250 hours.

There are often separate programs for people who want to train only as nail techs or electrologists, although these two programs are included in the full cosmetology program. To become a nail tech in California requires 400 hours, compared to 100 in Maryland and 250 in New York and Kansas. The electrologist program in California requires 600 hours of training. It is best to consult the school you are considering attending. Officials there will know the state requirements and have a program designed to meet them.

In addition to meeting state requirements for hours of training, all cosmetology school graduates must pass a state licensing exam before they can begin practicing their art. Again, each state establishes rules and regulations for its own licensing board. These requirements vary significantly across the United States, although some states recognize the training and licensing programs of other states in a system called reciprocity.

WHAT IT TAKES

Cosmetology is one of the leading careers in the personal service industry. When clients find a cosmetologist who is friendly, helpful, and skilled at making them look their best, a long and loyal relationship may be established. Ask around among your older friends and relatives. You are likely to discover individuals who have been visiting the same cosmetologist on a weekly or monthly basis for years, and who count this person as a friend.

In order to provide services tailored to clients' individual needs, a cosmetologist must know something about each person's lifestyle, career, and daily grooming regimen. This close working relationship generally leads to a bond of trust and friendship, prompting a feeling of loyalty on the part of clients. Such customers make standing appointments with a particular cosmetologist and may recommend that professional's services to friends and relatives as well.

In this way, a talented cosmetologist can develop a following of clients who provide job security and useful feedback. A loyal following can be very useful for a cosmetologist who decides to open his or her own salon—there will be guaranteed clientele from opening day on.

But what else does it take to make it as a cosmetologist? According to the National Cosmetology Association, success can be yours if you have certain personal qualities and characteristics. Ask yourself if you:

- Get along well with people
- Are artistically inclined
- Are willing to really listen to others
- Are dedicated to your career
- Have good health and stamina

Of course, much of your success will depend on excellent communication skills and the ability to put your own needs and desires aside while catering to those of the customer. In the course of a day's work, you may have to deal with a wide variety of clients, encountering people of all ages and dispositions. For the most part, they should be pleasant individuals, but there will be the inevitable client who is cranky, uncooperative, demanding, critical, or uncommunicative. It is the cosmetologist's job to maintain a friendly yet professional attitude, even when dealing with difficult personalities.

During your career, you can expect days when the services you perform are very repetitive in nature. There will be times when customers fail to show up for scheduled appointments. On occasion, you will need to deal with a disgruntled client whose perm did not take or who is consistently late for a scheduled appointment, thus affecting the balance of your day's schedule. Whether you own the shop or are the least experienced stylist working there, for the good of the business you will be expected to remain tactful, polite, and in charge of your emotions at all times.

You will need to have a high energy level. Hairstylists spend long hours on their feet. They also get their hands wet often, working with various shampoos, lotions, and other products that contain chemicals that may irritate the skin. For the most part, exposure to the fumes from various solutions used on the job is not a problem, although people with a history of asthma or allergies will want to consider this aspect carefully before choosing a career in the beauty industry.

A successful cosmetologist is drawn to a career in the beauty industry because of certain innate abilities, among them a strong sense of form, artistry, fashion, and creativity.

Because hairstyles are constantly changing, cosmetologists must keep up with the latest fashions and beauty techniques. This will require reading trade magazines or attending beauty trade shows. Your interest in a cosmetology career is sufficient to get you admitted to one of these extravaganzas, and the price of admission is often refunded through product purchases. These shows are fun, and for a few hours you will be able to immerse yourself a whole world of professional beauty care, checking out booths and displays showcasing the latest products and techniques. Some shows are limited to hair products, others to nail care. Many feature all aspects of cosmetology in a happy jumble. You will need a program to find your way around, pausing time and again to watch a platform artist at work or view a live product demonstration.

Managerial and business skills are important for those who plan to operate their own salons. A business owner needs the ability to judge a person's character, since hiring and managing a staff brings its own set of challenges.

INTERVIEW WITH A SUCCESSFUL COSMETOLOGIST
Meet Raina, a successful cosmetologist who agreed to offer advice to young people considering entering the field.

There's more to being a stylist than you realize when you first enroll in cosmetology school. But you figure that by the time you've accrued enough hours to take the state boards, you'll be ready. The problem is, you can know absolutely every answer on your tests, pass the state board exams, and still not have a clue how to do hair. The difference is experience. This is where the real learning begins. For instance, in the state board exam, you have to demonstrate how to make pin curls, but in reality, we don't use them. I've done finger waves, another part of the state exam, exactly zero times in my career. Even roller sets are becoming relics of the past.

Once you're at work in a salon, you suddenly have people asking what hairstyle will look good on them. You find yourself scrambling to remember what your instructors said about that in school. Something about round faces and square faces. Suddenly, you're terrified, wondering what in the world you're supposed to tell the client. So you grab a style book and try to get them to point to a picture that seems "safe," something you can do.

Then the next client sits down in your chair and wants a color. "Oh no," you're thinking, "she wants you to tell her what color would look best on her."

So you determine that she has cool undertones, or maybe they are warm . . . what was it you learned, anyway? I think it's the lack of experience that scares cosmetology school graduates in the early stages. It probably happens in every technical career. You've learned all this theory but haven't had much time to practice. It takes time to build confidence in yourself and your abilities. I hear more and more often of new stylists who get their license with no problem but leave the field in a short time. That's sad. Who knows how far these people could go, if only they had enough support and encouragement in the early stages. Good instructors are a key issue, in my opinion.

It takes years of experience in a salon to master the art, and cosmetology is an art. It's a continual learning process, since the tools and products we use are constantly changing.

WHAT TO EXPECT

As a rule of thumb, the less time it takes to train for a career, the more time it takes to get established on the job. This is certainly true of the beauty industry. A cosmetologist must be patient, working hard while getting established in the field. You may be sure that diligence will be rewarded. Typically, new graduates are given relatively simple assignments in the shop. After demonstrating their skills, they move on to more complicated tasks.

How you go about building a clientele varies from one salon to another. Many shops offer a two-tiered pricing schedule, charging a lower rate for services performed by the inexperienced staff members. Others assign new clients or walk-in customers to the less experienced stylists. By establishing your reputation for doing a good job and by building a good rapport with the clients you serve, you will encourage customers to ask for you when they schedule their next appointment.

Until a cosmetologist can build up a dependable client base or following, however, he or she may be paid a low hourly wage or a small income guarantee. For example, a newspaper classified ad seeking an entry-level hairstylist in a city of 350,000 persons offered a pay rate of just $5 per hour.

This will mean a restricted lifestyle for the first year or two. Still, a number of ads promised growth in skills and income for individuals who are committed to their careers.

As an example of what the experienced cosmetologist may expect in the way of job offers, here is how one salon described a vacancy for a hair technician:

Local salon currently seeking a personable, sensitive, reliable professional who wants to join an innovative team dedicated to excellent hair care. Opportunity for specialized training in a very rewarding, challenging career in a unique cosmetology service. Individual must possess a current state beauty operator's license, a valid driver's license, and a minimum of ten years' experience. Clientele not necessary. Excellent commission.

Cosmetologists enjoy their work, and this attitude is reflected in the way they talk about their careers. Don't be surprised at ads that describe a "fun staff" or "pleasant surroundings." Music, laughter, and an atmosphere of congeniality pervade most salons. When you are looking for work, be alert to the atmosphere that prevails in the shops you visit. You may come to think of the salon not only as your workplace, but also as a place where you can deal with people you care about and who trust your skills and abilities.

Even when you love your job, you will want an occasional vacation. Typically, salons provide at least a week's paid vacation, but there may be limitations on when you can take time off. For example, many shops are busiest during the summer months. The pace of work slows down in October, but picks up again in early December. Another slow period begins in mid-January, lasting until March. You may be asked to schedule your vacation during one of these periods.

Depending on the salon's operating schedule, employees may receive one or two days off per week. If you are in the habit of sleeping late on Saturday morning, better forget it—this is one of the busiest periods in a beauty salon's schedule. Except in some mall locations, most salons are closed on Sunday and Monday.

And what will you wear to work? Many salons have formal policies governing such issues as the style of dress and grooming for employees. Some require that all operators wear a uniform, perhaps a warm-up suit bearing the salon's name or logo. In others, the staff wear their own clothing. In summer, shorts may be permitted, but they are always conservative in length. The appearance and grooming of a salon's staff is a strong advertisement for the business. Hairstyles worn by the stylists should reflect the salon's best work.

OTHER DUTIES

For cosmetology school graduates, daily duties depend on the size of the business in which you are employed. In a small salon, cosmetologists may perform a variety of tasks on an as-needed basis, including scheduling appointments for clients, cleaning equipment, sterilizing instruments, and changing product displays or photographs that illustrate the latest hairstyles.

High standards of cleanliness and order are essential to the success of a salon. Even if the shop in which you work has a cleaning person who comes in at night, there will be cleaning tasks to perform throughout the day. You can expect to clean the station at which you work, sweeping the floor area after each haircut and sanitizing all combs and brushes. Between appointments, you will need to refill supplies at your work station and replace materials taken from the salon's supply room.

PRACTICAL EXPERIENCE

Because a cosmetologist must be licensed, it will be difficult for you to learn about this career without proper training, but many of the tools and materials a cosmetologist uses in the salon can be approximated at home. If friends and family are willing, you could see what it is like to cut and style hair, perform a manicure, even color or perm hair, using kits purchased in a health and beauty department of your local drugstore or beauty product store.

5

Choosing a School

Since your goal is to receive training that will prepare you to pass the cosmetology licensing exam, you should take care in selecting a cosmetology school. Accredited schools meet the standards of your state licensing board in such areas as instruction, modern equipment, and textbooks. They also balance their programs between classroom theory and clinical practice of the skills taught. Because many cosmetologists eventually become business operators, it would be wise to look for a school that also teaches such courses as basic bookkeeping, accounting, and sales techniques. Such topics are covered in accredited cosmetology schools.

Another important factor to consider when choosing a school is class size. An emphasis on hands-on training in a class of about twenty to twenty-five students is desirable, as are separate classroom facilities equipped for teaching and demonstrations of various techniques. During research for this book, cosmetologists repeatedly mentioned how important it is to receive individual attention from top-notch instructors. To succeed in this career, you need a combination of skill, charisma, and knowledge, best imparted by professionals who really care about their students.

Cosmetology training programs are offered in more than 3,500 public vocational and private training schools across the United States. To ensure the best investment of your training dollars, make sure that the school is accredited by the National Association of Trade and Technical Schools, which sets standards for the facility and its faculty. An important question to ask is what is the ratio of the school's graduates to those who obtain their cosmetology license. Also ask about the school's job placement program, since you will want to be involved with a program that assists you in getting your first job.

You may have a choice of attending classes during the day or in the evening. Some schools combine evening and Saturday classes, to accommodate students who are working their way through school. Those enrolled full time in a basic cosmetology course can expect to graduate in nine months to one year; then you will be prepared to take the state licensing exam for entry-level positions. Educational requirements vary from state to state, with some requiring as little as an eighth-grade education. Most states, however, require at least a high school diploma. A few states allow students to substitute an apprentice training program for graduation from a cosmetology school, but this is relatively rare. Details of two state apprenticeship programs are presented in this chapter. You should ask the schools' admissions directors for details on state requirements to practice cosmetology.

TOOLS OF THE TRADE

Cosmetologists use tools and equipment designed especially for this career. One of your first assignments in cosmetology school will be to learn the names of the tools, their functions, and learn how to care for them. You will use various types of scissors, razors, brushes, hair rollers, curling irons, blow-dryers, clippers, and massage and manicure equipment.

Early in your cosmetology training, you will acquire a professional tool kit. Some schools provide the necessary tools and equipment for your training. Others require that the students themselves purchase a kit of basic tools, including a case in which to transport them.

Priced at $650, a standard cosmetology kit consists of a carrying case and contents, including dual clips, a vent brush, three tail combs, a pair of shears, 12 dozen rollers with rack, a hair razor, a manicure kit, tapering shears, a sculptured nail kit, a 1/2-inch curling iron, a box of single-prong clips, a 3/4-inch curling iron, a shampoo cape, a nylon-bristle brush, two mannequins with stand, a blow-dryer, seven hairstyling combs, a back comb, and a hair net. Also included are a textbook, workbook, and exam book (one each) and six technical books on haircutting.

For those taking only the manicurist training, a student kit with textbooks is typically priced at about $300 and is likely to consist of a hard-shell carrying case containing various clippers, a disinfectant jar, emery boards, buffing blocks, a finger bowl, polish remover, nail strengthener, base coat and top coats, a hot oil heater, a maintenance kit, a metal pusher, an orangewood stick, a cuticle remover and nippers, a professional sculptured nail kit, textbook, workbook, and an exam review book.

Of course, the salon will also have certain fixtures for your use, including shampoo and dryer stations and reclining chairs. Most of the beauty supplies a stylist needs are supplied by the salon owner and are included in the client's bill for services. The shop may also include a cash register, a desktop computer, and a clothes washer and dryer, all of which the employees may be expected to operate. Perhaps you are surprised at the mention of laundry equipment, but according to an industry survey, the average beauty operator uses twenty-four towels per workday.

WHAT YOU LEARN
Your classes will be a combination of presentation methods relating to textbook reading assignments, audio-video material, lectures, and demonstrations of specific techniques. Increasingly, schools are making use of visiting artists or videotape presentations featuring internationally known stylists to supplement the classroom demonstrations provided by their own faculty.

Next, students begin hands-on training by practicing on mannequins and fellow students. As they gain experience, students get to work with salon customers who patronize the school's training clinic.

Cosmetology courses cover such topics as anatomy, basic physiology, hygiene, sanitation, job planning, applied chemistry, applied electricity, and cosmetology techniques. If you are seeking only a manicurist's license, the number of hours of necessary training is considerably less, and the cost of instruction is lower.

As the weeks go by, your instructors will be grading you on practical skills, personal and professional readiness, and academic performance. Of course, preparation for your career should follow a natural progression that allows you to master the techniques and skills of this art step-by-step. When your instructors assign you work with real customers in the school's salon, you will know that they recognize your growing competency in the art of cosmetology.

WHAT WILL BE REQUIRED OF YOU

Often, schools have a dress code and require that cosmetology students wear a uniform. Expect to deal with an attendance policy too. Most schools offer placement services for their graduates. This free help in locating a job is an important factor in selecting a school, since most salons fill vacancies by referrals from current employees, cosmetology school placement offices, and word of mouth.

Now let's get into the nitty-gritty of the courses you'll be taking. Remember that each state can set the required number of hours of instruction you must take in order to qualify for a manicurist or cosmetology license. What follows are examples of fairly typical requirements.

MANICURIST TRAINING

Manicurist training, a 300-hour program, prepares the student in all phases of professional manicuring and contemporary nail art/design. Once training and the state licensing exam are completed, the student will be ready for an entry-level position as a manicurist. Coursework covers theory, pedicuring, manicuring, sterilization, and hygiene. A manicurist license qualifies the graduate to apply artificial nails and perform manicures in beauty salons and barbershops. Tuition is generally around $1,500, plus the cost of the tool kit and uniform.

COSMETOLOGIST PROGRAM

Students can complete the operator-stylist program described here in approximately nine months. A breakdown of the topics covered follows:

- Professional practices—bacteriology, sterilization, sanitation
- Professional attitude—business practices and beauty culture law
- Sciences—histology (the study of tissue structure), trichology (the study of the structure, functions, and diseases of the hair), chemistry, physiology, cosmetic dermatology, electricity
- Cosmetology skills—shampooing, hair shaping, hair styling/finger waving, permanent waving, hair coloring, hair straightening, skin care, manicuring, temporary hair removal, scalp treatment, care of all hair types and textures

Studies include 1,250 hours of instruction and practice, which prepares students for the state licensing bureau examination and eventually prepares them to perform at entry-level jobs. Here is a list of typical programs, with the number of class hours noted: Theory, 200 hours; Finger waving/Hairstyling, 170 hours; Facials, 50 hours; Haircutting, 150 hours; Hair Coloring, 200 hours; Manicuring, 150 hours; Permanent Waving, 200 hours; Scalp Treatments, 50 hours; Shampoo/Rinses, 40 hours; Sterilization and Hygiene, 40 hours.

You may be familiar with the concept of competencies, that is, determinations of whether one's training meets a required level of accomplishment. The effectiveness of many cosmetology courses is now judged in this way. Some schools may use the following three-level competency list to measure student progress. Keep in mind that the student cannot progress to the next step until he or she has mastered every step in the previous level.

Students who have mastered Level One practice sanitation and sterilization procedures; give shampoos and different types of rinses; treat a variety of hair and scalp conditions; identify and describe skin and hair disorders; develop and display professional ethics, good grooming, and poise; demonstrate knowledge of a wide range of jobs and career options in cosmetology; do finger waving, perm wave wrapping, pin curls, eyebrow arching, and manicuring; perform massage; and provide skin care.

Students who have mastered Level Two can administer skin tests prior to applying tints and toners to clients; identify and describe anatomical and physiological systems; give a complete permanent wave; give a chemical hair relaxing treatment; apply tints, toners, highlighting, and pre-lightening; do marcel waving, hair designs, and various sets and comb-outs; and give a variety of facials.

Students who have mastered Level Three have acquired and can apply knowledge of theory to practicing beauty culture; they also know how to manage a salon and can pass the state board of cosmetology examination.

MASTER MANAGER PROGRAM

This is a 340-hour program (length varies from state to state) that prepares students to seek entry-level employment as a salon manager, after taking the state licensing exam. Course offerings include 100 hours in both business management and theory, plus 140 hours of class preparation/participation. Typical topics include: supervisory responsibilities, business management; health and public safety; and advanced hair coloring, restructuring, and cosmetology.

MASTER INSTRUCTOR PROGRAM

Students who wish to become instructors in cosmetology devote a total of 640 hours of study beyond that required for the cosmetology diploma. Remember that the required number of hours may vary from state to state. They must also take a state licensing exam for instructors. The course breakdown shows 100 hours of business management studies, 150 hours of theory courses, and 390 hours devoted to class preparation/participation.

Topics include theory and practical instruction, receptionist duties, dispensary (distribution of medications), managerial studies, operating the stock room, recruitment, and record-keeping.

COMBINED PROGRAMS

A number of schools offer combined programs, allowing students to build upon the basic foundation of their cosmetology training while acquiring additional skills as a master designer, master manager, or master instructor. Combined programs also allow for cross-over training, which enables a registered cosmetologist to become a registered barber, or vice versa.

Advanced training is also available to course graduates and licensed stylists who seek continuing education opportunities. Through a series of seminars and workshops, the working professionals receive instruction on new techniques and product knowledge from leaders in the cosmetology industry. International styling artists bring the latest trends and techniques to workshops via platform demonstrations.

A COSMETOLOGY CLASSROOM

Dana, a cosmetology school instructor, announces that today's lesson plan focuses on hair shaping, which is a skill cosmetologists use on a daily basis. Clients want more than an attractive haircut these days; they want a style they can maintain between visits to the salon. Hair shaping is the answer.

"This will be a basic scissors haircut," Dana announces to the group of students gathered in the school clinic. Six are seated in styling chairs, six are assigned to carry out the assignment. "Your first task is to assemble the necessary materials and equipment, using what you have learned from our previous work this week. You can begin."

Walking from one work station to the next, Dana makes note of the items each student has assembled for use. Her clipboard holds a checklist for each student, and she makes note of the items—client, clips, brush, spray bottle, towel, neck strips, comb, water, powder or talc, and a drape.

"The next step is to give the basic scissors haircut. Remember to section the hair as instructed earlier this week, and use the shaping techniques we have been practicing."

At each station, the student cosmetologist begins a quiet conversation with the client, seeking input on the style or effect he or she hopes to achieve. There is a certain amount of gesturing and demonstrating, as the stylist works to make sure he or she understands the client's expectations. One stylist steps away from her station long enough to secure a styling book, turning to a photo that she shows to her client.

"Yes," the client nods in agreement, "that's the look I want."

Five minutes into the exercise, all the clients have their hair pinned off in neat sections. Several of the students have begun using their scissors. Dana again makes the rounds of each work station, noting that stylists are cutting the required minimum half-inch of hair from all areas of the head, and checking that each student performed a scalp and hair analysis early in the procedure.

"I'm also checking that they use the implements correctly, and that when they have finished, the hair is blended uniformly. These items, along with proper draping of the client and correct use of sterilization techniques, complete this evaluation. Each student receives a copy of the evaluation form, which includes space for individual comments. We use a similar evaluation form for each module students demonstrate. There is also a multiple-choice test, given after the instruction but before the hands-on demonstration. Students who do not earn a passing grade on the written test do not proceed to working on a real head of hair until they repeat the module and pass the test."

YOU, THE STUDENT

From your first day in cosmetology school, you will sense an air of excitement. Every day will be different, filled with new experiences, new information, and the growing knowledge that you are becoming what you want to be—a skilled professional who is knowledgeable in the art and science of the beauty industry.

Since the safety and well-being of your clients is a prime consideration, your training will begin with this topic. You will learn about bacteriology, sterilization, and sanitation in terms of how they relate to salon operations. You will also learn how best to present yourself in the workplace, with discussions about hygiene and good grooming, visual poise, personality development, and professional ethics. Looking your best and presenting the best possible professional image are wonderful advertisements for your business—cosmetology.

Hair

Next comes the actual practice of cosmetology, where you will learn to drape the client to shield clothing from water, chemicals, and hair clippings. The proper technique for shampooing and rinsing comes next, and you will practice on fellow students. Scalp and hair-care topics follow, including scalp manipulation, dandruff treatment, and discussions on alopecia, commonly known as hair loss.

Once you have earned your scissors, so to speak, it is time to begin using those tools in hair-shaping classes. A combination of reading, lecture, and demonstration will precede any actual cutting on your part, and you will also learn how to section the hair for shaping and how to manipulate the necessary instruments. Such techniques as thinning and shingling along with the use of clippers and razor will be subjects for your practice. You will learn how to shape uncontrollably curly hair and how to deal with split ends.

After you've mastered the basic cut, it's time to develop even more finger dexterity and help prepare for the state board exams. You will learn horizontal, vertical, and alternate methods of finger waving as an introduction to the next topic, hairstyling.

Now you have been attending classes faithfully for several weeks. The opportunity to create hairstyles has your creative side fired up and ready for the next phase of your training. In addition to learning the professional way to remove tangles and make a part, you will also learn all the secrets of the pin curl—its parts, mobility, clockwise and counter-clockwise curls, how to shape and anchor them for various effects. Then you will move on to the ridge curl and the skip wave, graduating to the stand-up or cascade curl.

Now it's time to learn how to create volume and height with rollers and back-combing. You will also learn the important techniques involved in a good comb-out. Then you will learn how to take into consideration the varying degree of facial shapes and learn how to match them with the most flattering hairstyle.

As you continue to add to your store of knowledge, you will tackle such topics as long hair, permanent waving, body perms, and braiding.

And just when you really begin to feel comfortable working on clients, it's off to the wig salon, where you'll learn why people wear them, what they are made from, and how to care for and style them. In addition, you'll learn how they are made, how to order a wig to ensure a precise fit, how to set and comb-out a wig style—even change its color. And of course, falls, extensions, and hairpieces are included in this portion of your cosmetology training.

Think you're pretty handy with a blow-dryer? Wait until you work with a professional styling dryer, an invention of hairdressing guru Vidal Sassoon in London during the swinging 1960s.

Now that you are more confident with your newly acquired skills, it's time to enter a phase of your training that you might think of as Chemicals and the Cosmetologist. You'll get a chuckle from the history of the perm (especially the pictures) and come to appreciate the development of the "cold wave," which was so much quicker and more convenient for both customer and cosmetologist alike. Of course, to master this subject, you'll need to be alert and present in every class. After all, you'll be learning how human hair can be manipulated by chemical action, and your complete attention is necessary to learn safety rules and special problems. Successful cosmetologists will tell you that much depends on how expertly you wrap the hair and wind it on the curling rods.

Having mastered the perm, your next big challenge will be learning about hair coloring. If you have your heart set on the big time in cosmetology, becoming a skilled colorist is one sure route to the top. Expert knowledge of hair-coloring technique will provide you with a solid base of clients who will look to you for regular service for years to come. In addition to great job opportunities in the salon, a talented colorist can move up to work as a platform artist, manufacturer's representative, product consultant, and more. But you'll need a background in chemistry and computers, so be sure to pay attention when those topics are presented. Your cosmetology school days will focus on classifications of hair coloring, both lightening and darkening. You'll also learn about frosting, tipping, and streaking. When you learn about the business side of cosmetology, it will become immediately apparent that color services can make or break the salon.

Of course, by now you've tackled the subject of perms, but what about hair straightening? You'll learn about chemical hair relaxing and the thermal process. There are important techniques and products to use, and various approaches to hair of different lengths.

Since the licensed cosmetologist provides services beyond hair care, let's move on to the nails. Manicures and pedicures are our next subjects.

Nails

In today's busy business world, well-kept hands and nails are seen as a sign of good grooming, a dress-for-success detail not to be overlooked. From the cosmetologist's viewpoint, there is always the issue of health and safety to contend with. As part of your training, you will learn about nails and the various disorders that can affect nail health. Then you will become familiar with the tools of this trade and learn how to use them. Once you are comfortable at the manicurist's table, there will be a client on the opposite side, ready for you to perform a manicure. Of course, at first you will work on the hand model that is part of your manicurist's kit, moving on to fellow students as you gain expertise. You will learn about different shapes of nails and how to perform manicures simple and complex, on both women and men.

There are artistic aspects to manicures, and this may prove to be a special outlet for your creativity. It is at this point in their training that some cosmetology students choose a specialty, and some decide to become nail technicians. The lure of airbrushing and various other specialized nail design techniques brings out the artist in many. Before we leave this topic, you should know there are other skills to be learned, such as hand, arm, foot, and leg massages.

Skin

At some point in your training, you will be introduced to the work of an esthetician, or skin-care specialist. You will learn about facial treatments and makeup, from everyday cleansing to special spa treatments, including packs and wraps from mud to seaweed. You will learn the secrets of coordinating facial types with makeup technique to make the most of the client's natural good looks. You will enlist in the battle against wrinkles, learning about products and the art of concealing skin imperfections. There will be much to learn about daytime, evening, and theatrical makeup, and more opportunities to embark on a specialty field. Corrective makeup is another topic with far-reaching possibilities for you to explore.

Hair Removal

The topic of superfluous hair removal is quite fascinating. Superfluous means anything that is too much or not needed. The cosmetologist is trained to remove hair from the upper lip, the jawline, the arms, the bikini line—anywhere the client does not want it. There are temporary and permanent methods, from waxing to chemical depilatories and electrolysis, all of which you will be trained to perform. Permanent hair removal is a popular subsection of cosmetology and many choose to specialize in it.

Massage

Massage is another subject included in cosmetology training. The emphasis here is on the scalp, face, neck, shoulders, arms, and feet. You will learn the basic manipulations used in massage, along with the physiological effects created. Some of the topics discussed may include vibratory massage, joint movement, and the specifics of appliances used for facial and scalp massage.

Light Therapy

Let's also consider light therapy. You will learn how light rays are produced and how light therapy works to treat skin and scalp disorders and soothe body tissues with penetrating heat. You may have visited salons that offer tanning by ultraviolet light. Actually, there are many kinds of light rays, but cosmetologists are concerned with just three—those producing heat (infrared), those that produce chemical and germicidal reactions (ultraviolet), and visible light. All are natural elements of ordinary sunshine but have specialized uses in cosmetology. You will learn about therapeutic lamps, ultraviolet lamps, hot and cold quartz lamps, and their uses in cosmetology.

The Science of Cosmetology

No doubt you've been told there is some science to be learned en route to becoming a professional cosmetologist, and that is true. You will learn about histology, the study of cells, particularly skin cells and disorders of the skin. You will learn about tricology, the chemical makeup of hair and disorders of the scalp and hair. You will also study anatomy, particularly the head, shoulders, arms, hands, and feet. You will learn about bones, muscles, nerves, circulatory systems, and glands.

Regarding chemistry, your interest will be basically in those areas related to beauty products. The more you know about the chemical makeup of shampoos, rinses, permanent wave solutions, hair coloring, and cosmetics, the more skilled you will become as a cosmetologist. This knowledge may also form the foundation for career moves in your future. A number of executives in the beauty products industry work alongside learned scientists, yet do not have a college degree.

The Business Side of Cosmetology

And what about the business side of running a salon? Since the majority of cosmetology students have an interest in one day running their own salon, it is wise to choose a training program with a concentration in management. There will be instruction on planning the physical layout; hiring, training, and managing staff; sales aspects of the business; and day-to-day customer relations that will keep your business growing.

When your cosmetology instructors begin preparing you for the state licensing exam, you will know that your classroom time is coming to an end. The excitement of seeking and starting your first job now lies ahead. Those issues are addressed in chapters 6 and 7 of this book, but for now, remember that your days in cosmetology school are irreplaceable. Every successful cosmetologist interviewed for this book has stressed how important it is to attend every class and pay attention to every topic presented. Many credit their cosmetology training with giving them a start in their career, opening doors that led to surprising and rewarding opportunities, often without the need for a college background.

Specialized Schooling

With more than 1,000 accredited cosmetology schools operating across the United States, you are sure to find a program that suits your needs and budget. There are several schools that specialize in makeup artistry.

A school with a long history in this specialty is the Joe Blasco Makeup Academy, with locations in both Los Angeles and Orlando, Florida. The University of California, Los Angeles offers courses in makeup for film and television through its extension program. In nearby Toluca Lake is the Los Angeles School of Makeup Designory, offering a range of introductory to advanced courses. Then there is the Studio Makeup Academy, which is located inside a Hollywood film and television studio.

To learn more about these programs, contact the Admissions Director of the school:

Joe Blasco Makeup Academy
1670 Hillhurst Avenue, #202
Hollywood, CA 90027

Los Angeles School of Makeup Designory
10153 Riverside Drive
Toluca Lake, CA 91602
web site: www.makeupschool.com

The Studio Makeup Academy
1438 North Gower, Box 14
Studio 308
Hollywood, CA 90028
e-mail: studiomakeup@earthlink.net

It is not necessary for you go to California to learn about makeup for stage, screen, and photography. There are schools in New York State, Florida, Texas, the Great Plains, and many places in between.

What might you expect to learn in one of these programs? In general, the objective in theater makeup is to prepare students to provide makeup services for performing arts, including theatrical play productions, operas, ballet and dance recitals, musical and comedy groups, and nondramatic entertainment too.

Typically, you would take an introductory course covering the history of theater, stage lighting, and other working procedures in play production. Another course focuses on makeup designs for intimate, mid-, and long-range theaters—how close the audience is to the actors—known as intensity. Students also study makeup color, learning the importance of hue, value, and the effects of lighting on makeup.

Students also learn about specific makeup products: different brands, colors, and tools in stage makeup. Next are character studies designed to ensure that the makeup reflects the desired appearance of a character portrayed on stage. This course includes techniques for aging a character. Expect to learn about restructuring the face through the use of highlights and shadows, and disguises, using wax, putty, and false hairpieces.

Also taught are injury effects (bruises, cuts) and techniques for creating ethnic, comedic, and fanciful characters through makeup artistry.

Can You Afford Cosmetology School?

As we have already mentioned, vocational high schools are the bargain of the century, if you can make a career decision early in life. Those who have already graduated from high school can expect to invest $2,000 to $7,000 in becoming a cosmetologist. Scholarships, grants, and loans are available to help pay for school.

A new and valuable industry program is called ACE, which stands for Access to Cosmetology Education. Sponsored by the American Association of Cosmetology Schools, the Beauty Barber Supply Institute, and the Cosmetology Advancement Foundation, ACE scholarships are available across the United States. For details, call toll free (888) 411-GRANTS.

Manufacturers of beauty products also sponsor scholarship programs, and several private foundations make educational awards to promising cosmetology students.

6

The Licensing Exam and Beyond

Before you can launch your new career, you must secure a state license in cosmetology. To do so requires that you pass a state board exam, which all graduates of cosmetology programs must do. This consists of a written test and, usually, a practical test of cosmetology skills. Most states require that you recruit a volunteer model on whom you'll demonstrate haircutting or styling techniques, using your own tools and materials. In some states, an oral exam is included, and the applicant is asked to explain the procedures being following during the practical test.

While licensure requirements differ from state to state, in general, all states require that you be at least sixteen years of age and a high school graduate. Many states require that you pass a physical exam. State requirements for cosmetology instruction and practice range from approximately 1,000 to 2,500 hours. A separate test is given for those who seek only the manicurist license or a facial care license. The manicurist license requires from 200 to 350 hours of training, depending on the state.

Some states accept a license issued by another state without reexamination. You can check with a cosmetology school or state licensing board for details. Cosmetologists must renew their license every year (two years in some states) regardless of whether they have been working in their field. Should your license lapse, you will probably be required to take a refresher course of 40 hours or more before a new license is issued.

Toward the end of a course of study, many cosmetology schools include simulations to help prepare students for the state boards. Mock demonstrations, review sessions, and practice exams are typical activities. Don't worry; your instructors are well informed about the state exam and will make sure you have the information necessary to prepare for this experience. The best thing you can do is to listen attentively in class and practice the skills likely to be included in the practical test.

Cosmetology textbooks contain review questions, and practice tests are also available for the cosmetology boards in each state. A reference book entitled *Rudman's Questions and Answers on the Occupational Competency Exam in Cosmetology* is a frequently cited resource. The author is Jack Rudman, and the book is published by the National Learning Corporation in New York City.

Most states use a multiple-choice format on the written exam. A few still require hand-scoring of the written test, but many states offer same-day scoring of exams by an electronic scanner. You may well know your exam score before you leave the test site. All exams require a practical demonstration of skills, and some states include a face-to-face interview with an exam official, who questions the individual seeking a license. Usually, the state board exam is given in several locations at different times during the year, often within a month of graduation dates for cosmetology schools.

States charge varying fees for taking the state licensing exam and require that certain documents be presented at the time of testing. You will likely have to show at least one form of photo identification, plus proof of satisfactory completion of cosmetology training. The cosmetology license itself usually contains a photo ID.

Massachusetts is the first state to offer a daily walk-in service for both the practical exam and the electronic written exam. In this one-stop process, successful candidates receive their photo cosmetology license at the end of the testing session. This program has been so well received that other states are now looking at the Massachusetts program as a model.

PREPARING FOR THE WORKPLACE

The curriculum at many schools includes job-search workshops that teach students how to best present themselves during interviews. In such sessions, you will learn how to evaluate salons, and how to choose an environment that is right for you and your individual talents. There is also a book by Victoria Harper entitled *Professional by Choice: Milady's Career Development Guide*, designed to help cosmetology students get established in careers.

If your cosmetology school sponsors a chapter of the Future Cosmetologists organization, consider membership as an active or associate member. In addition to hosting hair and beauty shows at the local level, this club will help you make professional contacts. The club also has a job placement component.

INTERNSHIPS AND APPRENTICESHIPS

Some schools combine formal training with an internship in a licensed salon. This is where you get actual work experience while you study. Although most interns are not paid for their services, they often receive class credit or some other kind of professional recognition. The most important thing earned in an internship is how to best ply your craft.

The apprenticeship approach to learning a trade has a long history, and it is gaining renewed attention as young people examine alternative ways to gain job skills. In a cosmetology apprenticeship, the student is responsible for finding a mentor—that is, a licensed cosmetologist, willing to hire the would-be cosmetologist for minimal wages in exchange for learning by doing. Most programs require apprentices to work a certain number of hours, covering a period of one to three years. Many states do not issue a license for skills learned by apprenticeship. States that do recognize apprenticeship as a method for learning cosmetology maintain strict conditions for the training. Wisconsin and Idaho are among the states that have apprenticeship programs in cosmetology. To find out whether your state offers one, contact the state licensing board.

Besides giving you hands-on experience, internships and apprenticeships are also excellent sources of networking. Contacts you make during these training periods could help you land a job, perhaps in the very salon where you had your internship or apprenticeship.

UNIONS AND PROFESSIONAL ORGANIZATIONS

Not many cosmetologists belong to a labor union, but those who do are represented by the United Food and Commercial Workers International Union. Its membership includes both salon owners and employees.

7

Entering the World of Work

As previously mentioned, there is no shortage of jobs out there. The challenge will be finding the job that is best for you.

It is quite likely that you will be receiving offers before you graduate, if your attitude is good and you are developing professional competencies. Of course, you will need to pass your state's cosmetology licensing exam before you can begin working professionally.

In our previous discussion about choosing the right cosmetology school, we touched on the importance of an active job placement service. Most placement services concentrate on a radius of about fifty miles. What if you want to work outside the immediate area served by your cosmetology school? If so, you may have to do some work on your own to find the right first job.

No matter where you work, you will want to develop a career ladder, making sure that your position increases in rewards and responsibilities as you move upward through the ranks.

SOURCES FOR FINDING A JOB

Previously we discussed how placement programs, internships, and apprenticeships can help cosmetology graduates find jobs. There are other sources that can also help you enter the workforce. Newspaper classified sections and the Internet are excellent sources for cosmetologists. In addition to learning what sorts of jobs are available, you can learn what salon owners are looking for in new employees. What follows are sample ads from both sources, newspapers first:

HAIR DESIGNERS—Need 2 talented professionals NOW! Guaranteed $7.25 an hour base + commission. Average $9-14 per hr. Benefits avail. Paid vacations, no employment contract required. Two suburban mall locations.

HAIR DESIGNERS, MANAGERS, AND MANICURISTS—Experienced, coming back to the industry, or a recent graduate? Our salons have a position for you! Get paid for your experience. You can earn up to $15 an hour or more, plus product commission and a $1,500 advancement bonus. Salon managers are paid salary and salon bonus. Medical, life, profit sharing and vacation benefits, plus free advanced training. Call for an appointment, or visit one of our salons at these (10) downtown and suburban locations.

COSMETOLOGY INSTRUCTORS—Full-time and part-time positions in our two community college locations. Teacher's license required.

HAIRSTYLIST/MANICURIST—Part time, hourly wage or 50-55-60 commission, your choice. Paid vacation.

And now, from the Internet. The next two postings are excerpted from the bulletin board maintained by the

National Accrediting Commission of Cosmetology Arts and Sciences (NACCAS) in Arlington, Va. The address for this Internet site is: http://www.naccas.org. Another Internet source of job information is called Spa/Salon Staffing at http://www.beautytech.com. This site offers a national employment registry for cosmetologists, which is updated each month. The remaining listings come from the home page of a chain of salons based in Seattle. Similar information is available from various Internet search engines.

SHOP MANAGER—$18-20,000 salary, bonus up to $7,000 annually. Minimum 2 yrs. experience with proven ability to grow sales. Duties include setting the example as a stylist, administration, staff training, and development plus recruitment. We offer a fair and principled work environment. Benefits include medical, dental, vision, paid vacations and holidays, personal days, ongoing and free training, and opportunity for advancement. Position is in Tampa, Fla.

INSTRUCTOR—Esthetics and massage at a Chicago area school. Position requires 24-32 hours per week. Prior work and educational experience in cosmetology a plus.

ASSISTANT MANAGER—Uses company's technical system to provide quality haircuts and perms; provides excellent customer service; recommends/suggests product purchases to customers; promotes and maintains high standards of quality in the salon; assists in salon management and supports manager in all areas; maintains equipment and reinforces salon cleanliness and appearance; keeps accurate customer records.

STYLIST—Seeking individual with cosmetology license, excellent customer-handling skills; flexible schedule, efficient manner and willingness to learn; ability to represent and explain products offered in shop; skillful in handling customer complaints and re-dos, if necessary; neat, tidy, skilled in performing cuts and perms. We offer competitive pay, health insurance, paid vacations, and direct deposit of paychecks.

HAIRDRESSERS AND MANAGERS—Sought for chain salon with locations in Phoenix, San Francisco, Los Angeles, and Ohio locations.

NAIL TECH—resort at Grand Cayman Island.

YOUR RÉSUMÉ

You probably know that a résumé is a written summary of your education, training, and work experience. Most students have written at least one by the time they graduate from high school. There are different types of résumés for different situations, but the basic information should be scrupulously accurate, restricted to one page, and printed on paper designed for résumés. White or off-white paper makes the most professional impression.

When you are seeking work, keep your résumé up-to-date, making sure there are no misspelled words and that the document is representative of the best work you can produce. Every time you make a contact, visit a salon, or meet someone who could help you get the job you want, ask if you may leave a copy of your résumé.

As part of a formal job-seeking, your résumé should be accompanied by a cover letter, briefly explaining your career goals for the next five years and stating your willingness to interview for the job. It's not necessary to go into detail about your training or experience, since that information is in the résumé. Be sure your name, address, and contact information are clearly stated, and sign the cover letter in your best penmanship. Use a pen with black or blue ink to sign the letter.

THE JOB INTERVIEW

Once your letter and résumé have met with approval, it's time to meet face-to-face. Most hiring decisions rely heavily on the results of a job interview. This may involve one or more meetings between the candidate (you) and the salon owner or manager.

It is natural to feel a bit nervous before a job interview. A little preparation will boost your self-confidence and help you make the best possible impression on the interviewer. There are several ways to prepare yourself for the interview experience, some of which will be covered in the closing weeks of your cosmetology course work.

Start by knowing about the specific job you want and the business in general. During the interview, you should ask some questions too. Your questions should also reflect initiative, another positive trait. If you sit in silence or fumble for an answer when the interviewer asks a question, you will probably lose points. Topics you can inquire about include the job duties, working conditions, the qualifications required for the particular job, and opportunities for advancement. Other questions might involve the availability of fringe benefits and typical work schedules for the salon.

Your cosmetology course may include mock job interviews. If not, you can still prepare by anticipating some of the questions the interviewer may ask of you, including:

- Why do you want to work at this salon?
- Why do you think you are qualified for this job?
- Tell me about yourself and the work you like to do.

As part of the interview process, you may be asked about your family, how you spend your spare time, what you think you might be doing in five years, what you consider to be your major strengths and weaknesses, or the subjects you liked best in school. To prepare, put your thoughts on paper. Practice a response for each question until you can say it aloud and feel comfortable doing so. Be sure your response is genuine and shows something about who you really are. All the while, remember to emphasize your strengths; don't forget to admit your weaknesses (though you can downplay them). Remember that making direct eye contact is important.

Of course, you always want to be properly groomed—after all, you represent the beauty industry. On the day of your interview, be sure you've had a good night's sleep. Arrive a few minutes early, and wear attractive, yet appropriate business attire. Don't smoke in the reception room or during the interview, even if invited to do so. When someone approaches to greet you, stand and offer to shake hands, whether the individual is male or female. Remember to smile and be friendly.

Carry whatever documents you plan to submit in an envelope or clip them inside a folder. Make sure your name, address, and phone number appear on every page. Don't shuffle through your paperwork.

During the interview itself, remember to look the person in the eye, which is not to say that you should stare. Lean forward a little bit and demonstrate that you are a careful listener. Don't fidget. An occasional gesture is fine; otherwise keep your hands folded in your lap or resting quietly on the arms of your chair. Your voice should be clear and assertive in tone. Remember, your communication skills are an important part of the job you will be doing. Above all, don't complain about past instructors or employers. Sometimes this is a trap that is deliberately set by potential employers.

Don't be surprised if you are asked to demonstrate some practical skill as part of the interview. Stylists have been asked to do a comb-out, nail techs to apply nail tips or a coat of lacquer.

At the close of the interview, shake hands again. Most interviews end with a noncommittal comment such as "Thanks for coming in," or "We'll get back to you soon." You may leave with no idea how you did or whether you have a chance at being hired. While it takes a bit of time and effort, it is still wise to send a brief follow-up note to the interviewer, thanking him or her for meeting with you and again mentioning your interest in the job. Do not ask whether you got the job; simply say thanks and make sure your full name, address, and phone number are in the message. Mail the note the day after the interview. It is a surprisingly effective move, as employers will remember your good manners and communication skills.

Should you simply wait for a phone call? If you have not heard within a week or so, it is acceptable to call the interviewer. Simply ask about the status of the job. Has the position been filled? Are you still being considered? If not, it's time to apply elsewhere. Even if you don't get the first job you apply for, going through an interview is a valuable experience that will help you relax and feel more confident the next time.

THE PORTFOLIO

As you near the end of your professional training, ask one or two of your instructors for a written recommendation stating your particular strengths as a cosmetologist. Photocopy these documents and include them in an interview packet with your cover letter and résumé. Some employers may even request these letters of recommendation.

You may also want to compile a portfolio of photos that illustrate your best work, which you can show to a prospective employer during an interview. Include a few photos of yourself in action, actually performing a manicure or cutting hair.

Some enterprising job seekers have set up video cameras in the salon, taping their interaction with clients as well as capturing their cosmetology skills in living color. Copies of the tape are included in their interview packet. Of course, you will need the permission of your client before filming. Also, don't assume that the salon at which you are interviewing will have a VCR available. Mention during your interview that you have the tape with you. If the interviewer expresses interest, offer to leave a copy (not the original) and arrange to pick it up at a later date.

8

Meet the Pros

Now it is time to meet some professionals in the world of cosmetology. Some of these names you may recognize, others are introduced by first name only, but all are professionals at various stages of their careers in the beauty industry. From student to seasoned salon owner, their experiences are typical of the business in the United States. In every case, interview subjects were willing and eager to tell it like it is.

A COSMETOLOGY STUDENT

At age nineteen, Eline is midway through the training course at a long-established career academy. The school trains people in several technical fields, although the cosmetology program draws the largest enrollment. The fully certified program includes classes in which the student-to-instructor ratio is 20 to 1, and the academy's clinic draws a wide range of clients—from the senior citizen apartment complex in the neighborhood to the university housing a few blocks away.

Asked what sparked an interest in cosmetology as a career choice, Eline explains:

> *I was always the one at the end of gym class French-braiding a friend's hair. In fact, I was also always the one who had to dig through a backpack full*

of combs, hairsprays, and mousse in order to find my notebook or a pen. When I went to the library to take notes on current events for history class, I'd find the news magazines and start looking up current events, but then I'd find myself distracted by the pictures—I was always more interested in the hairdos and clothing styles.

How do beauty school classes differ from regular high school classes?

They are more fun, definitely more fun. We get to see what the instructor is doing up-close, and hear a step-by-step description too. Then we try the techniques ourselves. We each have a lab partner and take turns being the stylist or client.

The instructors really care about our progress. They have instant cameras in class and take photos of the best work, which they display on a bulletin board in the reception hall. This shows off your work not only to students, but to the clients who come to our school salon. It's really great when someone asks for you personally based on something they've seen in a photo.

These instructors always stress professionalism, in both work and attitude. You have to be the kind of stylist that people like, so they'll ask for you for their haircut, perm, or whatever.

I think I'd like to specialize in children's haircuts. I get along well with little kids. My reflexes are quick, so if the child moved suddenly, I could adjust the clippers or scissors and not ruin the job. Of course, a child's haircut is the least expensive service in a salon, so that makes me think twice. There are days when I think specializing in hair coloring is the way to go. I love to mix tints and match them to the palette of facial tones. The school encourages us to experiment with color. I've had highlights glazed in all summer, and I'm thinking about trying a soft, golden blonde for fall. My lab partner has light brown hair and wants to try some reddish highlights.

It's great to understand how tints combine and what you can do with them. The unit includes work in color corrections too. For example, if someone has made a mistake, usually with a home coloring kit, and turned her hair green or something. We learn to take her back to her normal color without damaging her hair.

When asked what she will do to find her first job, Eline's immediate response is:

Oh, I've already started looking. One of the reasons I chose this school is because of its placement office. They get calls all the time from salon owners and managers looking for the school's top graduates, or people who really stand out in one skill or another. To motivate those of us who still have a way to go before being hired, the office posts the job descriptions they are asked to fill. We meet the school's graduates who come as guest artists, and they tell us what it's like in the working world.

I want my first job to be in the city, at one of the salons where they do high-fashion cuts and hairstyles. After a few years, I can see myself going back to the area where I grew up and running my own salon. I want to own my own home and have a family, so a cosmetology business makes a lot of sense. When I start a family, I can hire someone to take my place as manager for six months at a time, and I can just do the books at home.

Yes, I've heard all those tales about how tough it is to get started. That's why I concentrate on building my salesmanship skills and communication with clients. I want to make a good first impression, provide the best service possible, and please the customers. If I have to, I'll share an apartment with roommates and take the bus to work or eat brown-bag lunches for as long as it takes. I'm lucky not to owe money for my education.

OWNER OF A THRIVING SALON

The salon is decorated with red and black graphic designs on a soft gray-white background, a sort of industrial look with metal shelving and exposed pipes. The reception area is full, and two clients are booking their next appointments. Both manicurists are at work, and a stylist is demonstrating hair-care products to yet another client as cool jazz wafts from stereo speakers. This business is obviously prospering.

"Right now, I could use another stylist," says David, owner of this five-chair salon. "Someone who handles a razor with confidence and has a sense of style, that's who I'd like to meet."

David made a major life change five years ago. "I'd been interested in cosmetology in high school, but my guidance counselor and parents talked me out of it, so I went into banking instead. A few years later, a relative enrolled in cosmetology, and when we talked about the training, I realized my interest was still there."

Several factors worked in David's favor. Motivation

was high on the list, as was the backing of a supportive spouse. As an adult student with a family to support, David knew this career change had to be a success, thus motivating him to work diligently in class.

"We were using our savings to pay for my schooling, and the family budget took a wrenching, going down to one income for most of a year. I wanted to prove it would all be worth the sacrifice and risk. The payoff was the chance to do work I wanted, to take a risk and have it pay off."

David did so well, in fact, that the academy's instructors recommended that he join them on the teaching staff a year after he had graduated. He subsequently added a teacher's license to his training.

In fact, within five years of leaving his job as a bank manager, David had completed cosmetology school, worked as a hair stylist, been named director for a chain of salons, and was contemplating going into business on his own.

"My experience proves that you don't need to worry about hitting a dead end in this career. Everything depends on your ability and what you want to accomplish."

David purchased the business from someone who was ready to retire. He took over the lease in a commercial building convenient to parking and an office building where hundreds of potential clients worked.

"The price included a fee for 'goodwill,' the value of the equipment and the inventory. It's hard to put a price on goodwill, but an accountant helped in working out that part. The goodwill consisted of the client records, the former owner's time spent training me during the transition in ownership, and a week of endorsing my skills and competence to existing clients."

David also comments on the modern technology he uses to help his salon run smoothly.

"We use a computer to keep track of many salon details, including what services were rendered during every client visit. We take note of things like formulas for hair coloring, perm solutions, the number of weeks elapsed since the last cut, any changes that were made, that sort of thing. It's also an excellent way to keep track of inventory and monitor our use of supplies. Of course, it also simplifies bookkeeping, ordering, and handling the payroll. You can see which operators are doing a lot of cuts, which are giving a lot of perms, and so on."

Computer-generated images are now being used in some salons to preview the way a client would look with various hairstyles, colors, and cuts. Such systems, however, can cost upwards of $10,000, and are appearing first in highly competitive metropolitan areas. "Of course, I'd love to have the computer imaging program, but it's a few hundred cut and dye jobs from reality just now," David laughs. "I've seen the system demonstrated at hair shows, and I understand that the big chains that are into full-scale beauty consultations are using them. I know my clientele, and they are not ready for the extra cost. But you know how these computer programs come down in price once the novelty begins to wear off. Who knows, maybe in a year or two, I will be able to afford it."

Because the business has seasonal peaks and valleys in terms of volume, the owner does not always receive a weekly paycheck. "It depends on the cash flow. I have to pay operating expenses and suppliers and the payroll. Those things come first. I know when money's there, and I take what I need."

Reluctant to offer specifics on income, David pointed out that both of the senior stylists on his staff had bought their own homes in the past two years, and the manicurist had just bought a new car.

"My older child has just started college, and I expect to send the younger one in two years. I figure my situation is about the same as most business owners in this community. I can afford some time off, but making the time is the hard part."

There has been no reason to regret leaving the banking industry. In fact, the bank where this individual had worked went through a series of mergers, resulting in the elimination of an entire department. Ironically, it was the department David had worked in.

Asked whether there was one aspect of the training or job that came as a surprise, David responded, "Yes—the funeral home visit." After five years in the business, David was called on by the family of a long-term client. Luckily, as part of their training, all would-be cosmetologists tour a mortuary, including the preparation room.

"They wanted her hair to look like it always did, and figured the way to accomplish that was by having the person who always did the set and comb-out take care of it one last time."

Does he have advice to newcomers in the beauty industry?

"Just remember that service means everything in this industry. It can literally make or break your salon. Craft counts, certainly, but so much of the clients' decision to return is based on their treatment. Did the client get what he or she wanted? Was the service personalized? How well did your staff communicate with him or her?

"Everyone involved with your shop must continually remind themselves to go that extra step in service. That means knowing something about the client's lifestyle—how much time she has to care for her hair. But it also means using a little bit of psychology too. You need to greet the customer, keeping the social interaction and the service you're performing on track. It's important to have the client's input with every step, but you must have clear communication going in both directions. Sometimes the client is interested in a change, something a little bit different. This often happens in January, after the holidays when people are feeling a little bored with the routine. A new hairstyle can lift a mood, change thinking, or attract a little attention to the wearer. This is where the link between looking good and feeling good about oneself comes into play.

"The client who feels he or she received personalized service will develop a loyalty to your salon, recommending it to friends and family. That's what success is all about."

While it is a career that starts out slowly and demands long hours and excellent communication skills, cosmetology offers many rewards and challenges.

Would David recommend that one of his children follow in the path of his career choice?

"Definitely; I'd recommend it for either one."

Meet a Nail Technician

I am a nail technician; that means a manicurist specially trained to apply and decorate artificial fingernails.

In a week, I may see 80 to 100 clients, some of them for the first time, others who have been my clients for years. When prom and graduation times come up, I am especially busy, because women want to maintain a high level of grooming and a certain level of elegance for these formal occasions.

Basically, I view my work as having two phases: first I create dramatic nails where there were none; then I decorate those nails in artistic ways.

I really love to work with paints and the airbrush. I keep up-to-date on new ideas and sketch some original designs of my own, which I display in my workplace, using artificial press-on nails as my canvas, if you will—seasonal themes, personalized designs, anything that catches my fancy, really.

Much of the work is accomplished with decals these days, and many of my clients have developed a real signature look with, say, a star that they use on the corner of an eyeglass frame, in their earring or jewelry design, and also in their manicure. For others, it's a signature color that is repeated in several ways. My clients think of their nails as accessories, and frankly, once they've got them, they don't mind flaunting them a little. I get a lot of new business through referrals.

I spend a fair amount of time educating my clients about how to take care of their nails, especially if the look is new for them. I tell them, "Treat your nails like jewels, not tools." They should really be coming in about every two weeks for maintenance, but at first, there is often repair work until the client learns to avoid damage or breakage. The biggest risks come from opening pop-top soda cans, dialing the phone, and lifting heavy objects. All of these put upward pressure on the tips of their nails, and the material is not designed for it.

I also work hard to keep my clients aware of allergic reactions to acrylic products. It's rare, but it can happen. I want them to call in as soon as they notice any abnormal condition of the nail.

Likewise, in my studio, I am absolutely meticulous about sanitation. I use a hospital grade disinfectant and disposable tools whenever possible. Antibacterial soap and good hand washing are part of our routine between each and every service. What are we being so careful about? There are several issues here, but cosmetologists are particularly concerned about safety and disease transmitted via body fluids, including the AIDS virus. It's not smart to ignore it. Dentists take precautions for themselves and for their patients; so do cosmetologists.

My best advice to clients? If you wash dishes, have a good pair of rubber gloves and give your hands and nails a beauty treatment while washing. Apply cuticle oil and/or hand lotion that does not contain mineral oil—that will lift acrylic nails—and wear the gloves while you wash up after dinner. The heat of the dishwater helps the skin absorb lotion or oil. It's also a form of hand exercise and is quite soothing.

NAIL TECH NUMBER TWO—A DIFFERENT ANGLE

I worked my way through college as a manicurist. When I became an advertising executive, my first project was in the beauty products industry. We're trying to anticipate market trends and be ready to launch new products successfully.

We've been in the photo studio all week, preparing for a print campaign using close-up shots of the new colors. That means working with hand models. These are people who make a living having their hands photographed. You know, long, slender fingers and no calluses or bumpy knuckles. Their nails are exquisite too, as you might imagine. The manufacturer sends two very talented manicurists to the studio for every session, and the models go through a series of shots wearing the different polishes. Sometimes both hands are done with the same product, sometimes every finger is a different shade, to showcase an entire line.

To everyone else, it's just the start of spring, but with magazine and TV ad deadlines such as they are, we're thinking about autumn in this campaign. The colors are dark, tending toward browns, with lots of metallic and mica accents.

And there's something else that's new. Nail polish for men. Not just a couple of coats of clear lacquer with a manicure, but colors, too.

The target audience is an age group from twelve to thirty years. I understand the marketing director on this project asked her husband to try the colors when he wore sandals. He liked the look so much, he's still using a color called "Sand." Will men in their forties pay $12 for a bottle of nail polish? It will be interesting to find out. A half-dozen leading department stores are carrying them now.

I still use my manicurist kit, but only for myself and family members, at no charge. I like being ahead of the pack in nail fashion, but even more, I get a thrill out of opening a new magazine issue and seeing my new campaign in living color.

HAIR COLOR SPECIALIST

Speaking of color, our next interview is with a hair color specialist on the Pacific Coast. Mark, who owns the salon, is proud to be a "team player," at work in a salon where color is everyone's specialty, and the team spirit prevails, since competition for clients is minimized.

Our salon opened in this location nearly fifteen years ago, with just three stylists. Within five years, it expanded to include the space next door, and now it's 3,000 square feet of space, where twenty-four of us work on a full- or part-time basis. Our clientele is primarily upscale, ranging in age from late twenties to early sixties. Most are female, but about 15 to 20 percent of the people we see for cuts, texture, or color services are men.

Many of our clients are interested in great hair color, which happens to be our specialty. Our primary concern is superior customer service. Every member of the staff is expected to meet the same list of competencies, which means that any client can work with any team member. The use of computer records to track each client's history with the salon helps make this program workable.

How does the team approach benefit clients?

From the client's point of view, the team approach helps eliminate the frustration of a waiting list, something clients of other salons encounter when they make appointments with their stylist. If you color your hair, you know that regular maintenance can't wait, it needs to be done on schedule to keep the color looking good and avoid problems with new growth at the hair's roots.

Of course, the system requires that lines of communication be open regarding client information, and that we maintain a close-knit environment within our staff. We are able to do this because we have very little turnover. Staff members like the system; they are able to earn a good living, regardless of their seniority here; and all have as many bookings in a day as they want to handle. The teamwork approach pays dividends in many ways.

Our stylists pride themselves on their professionalism, and in turn, management rewards them by giving them the opportunity to reach their full potential. The salon itself is a beautiful working environment, with an atmosphere that is supportive and friendly. At our weekly team meetings, the focus is on cooperation, a unified purpose, and high morale. We are not only a team, but a group of artists who appreciate the value of education. We are always learning and improving.

What kind of clients come to your salon?

The clients we serve come from all over Silicon Valley. They are attracted to our neighborhood, which has a certain European atmosphere. In addition to upscale beauty services, there are interesting shops and restaurants nearby. Clients often make a day of it: having their hair done in addition to visiting the other attractions in the area.

What makes the success of your salon possible?

Our reputation for color services is undoubtedly what brings in many of our new clients who have been referred to us by their friends. The revenue they generate keeps the salon growing.

One thing feeds on another, in a positive way. The reliable revenue flow makes possible a training program that is ongoing and extensive. We use a four-level certification program for staff skills, beginning with bronze and working up through platinum. It covers the facets of technical, professional, and interpersonal skills. Then we help finance advanced education at the leading academies, including Vidal Sassoon, Bumble & Bumble, and Toni & Guy. As staff members complete education modules, they are tested and advance to the next level. Of course, compensation reflects these increasingly sophisticated skills.

We move our new team members from straight salary to a structured base plus commission system. Commissions are calculated not only on production, but also on educational progress and on meeting preset objectives—customer service skills and client retention are tops on that list. Our team philosophy extends to a profit-sharing plan, in which incentive bonuses are earned through team accomplishments.

The team approach also spills over into business aspects of the salon as well.

Employees play an active role in the financial management of our company through the "open book" process. They know how well the business is doing, if they care to look at the records. Team members have a direct effect on the bottom line and can also influence the amount of money that goes into their pockets. There are other perks involved with working at this salon.

We offer health-care benefits. After six months on the team, full-time staff members receive a 50 percent contribution to a health maintenance organization. Other benefits include a paid vacation of five days in the first year, and seven days in the second year. After three years, staff receive two weeks off with pay. Part-time staff earn vacation that is prorated, depending on the number of hours worked.

Asked what type of person he is looking to hire, Mark responds:

The beauty industry is customer-driven, which is the basic reason we look for new staff members who are looking for an environment in which they can grow and develop their potential over the long term. We want people who are excited by change and eager to learn new techniques. Our recruitment program begins with a résumé and cover letter. We receive them in the mail almost daily, but we also encourage people to stop in and deliver a résumé in person.

MEET AN ELECTROLOGIST

Marianne is a licensed, board-certified hypertrichologist.

In short, that means I am professionally trained in the safe and permanent removal of unwanted facial and body hair. I am an active member of my home state's Hypertrichologist Association, as well as the American Electrology Association, and I mak an effort to keep up-to-date on the latest developments in this industry.

Marianne's location is a little different from that of an average salon.

For the convenience and privacy of my clients, I maintain an office in my home, offering flexible hours during the day, the evening, and on Saturdays. I work by appointment only—no walk-ins. The business is located in an addition to the original house, with a separate entry and a suite of treatment rooms down the hall from the office and reception area. The emphasis here is on privacy and a peaceful, relaxed atmosphere.

I like the fact that there is no commute to work, and the nature of this business does not detract from a residential neighborhood in any way. The lots are large, and since there are rarely more than three clients here at one time, parking is not an issue.

In building a clientele, Marianne sees many people who are new to the procedure.

Many of our clients come in for their first visit seeking information before they make a decision about electrolysis. We offer a complimentary consultation and sample treatment. Our goal is to provide the highest level of comfort and effectiveness.

The service I provide uses electrolysis for the permanent and safe removal of facial and body hair. Both men and women use our services. The equipment here is state-of-the-art. Complete sterilization and sterile, disposable probes are used. In addition, three methods of electrolysis are available. These methods are tailored to each individual's comfort level and hair type to achieve maximum results. The electrolysis is performed by trained professionals who have met or exceeded the strict licensing requirements of this state.

Marianne's electrolysis business grew as the result of training and her experiences at other jobs.

I received my first training in this field while earning my cosmetology license. Over the years, electrolysis became something of a specialty, to the point where I had very little time for hairstyling. Some electrologists work in beauty salons or at day spas. I've done both, but when I decided to open my own business, I made a decision to focus just on electrolysis.

At first, I was the owner, manager, and only employee. Now I have two part-time workers who help take care of the evening and Saturday workload. We've added a line of skin-care products, but that's about the extent of our merchandising.

Is electrology painless?

Well, first of all, let's use the term discomfort. And it varies from person to person, depending on individual thresholds. It also depends on the part of the body where the unwanted hair grows. For most, the upper lip is the most sensitive area. Generally, legs and forearms are the least sensitive parts. Most people feel only a tingling sensation. Likewise, the number of treatment sessions and the length of these sessions varies according to the individual.

Our sessions last from fifteen to sixty minutes, determined by three factors: the type of hair follicles, previous types of hair removal used by the client (primarily waxing and tweezing), and the client's general health and well-being.

Are there any extra precautions you take in your line of work?

Yes, we carry professional malpractice insurance. And, yes, there are areas where an electrologist is not permitted to remove hair: the mucous membranes, such as the nostrils, and hair growing from moles, unless the client brings in written permission from a physician. Even then, many states have laws prohibiting treatment involving moles, or insurance policies forbid it.

Perhaps it would be more clear to discuss areas where we can remove hair: from the upper and lower lip, chin, cheek, hairline, or neckline. We may also thin or remove the hair from a beard, the bridge of the nose, where eyebrows grow in a straight line, and from the back and arms, legs and chest.

The actual technique sounds rather simple, but it takes diligence and practice to master it. Poor technique can result in a skin surface that looks pitted. Certainly, you want to avoid that result. Hair follicles are quite small, so the work site is viewed through an illuminated magnifier. Some electrologists choose to wear magnifying glasses instead. You hold the probe in one hand and gently manipulate the skin with the other. I want to emphasize that there is no puncture of the skin. That remains a nagging misconception about electrolysis. Instead, a very fine wire is inserted into the opening of the hair follicle itself. A tiny amount of electric current passes from the probe to the papilla, the tissue that feeds the hair root, and disables it, stopping hair growth.

Everything about this equipment is carefully calibrated to use the smallest amount of current necessary to accomplish the goal. Electrologists are well trained in adjusting the timing and intensity of the current. There are also timing circuits built into the equipment as an additional safeguard for clients.

My equipment is controlled by a foot pedal. There is no pulling of the hair. We use fine forceps to slide out the detached hair. The essential skill is the precise insertion of the probe, every time, and for every hair follicle.

What skills are necessary to be a successful hypertrichologist?

Obviously, good vision and steady hands are important in performing this work. You also need patience, as sessions may last from fifteen minutes to an hour. It is exacting and sometimes tedious, repetitive work.

You need some psychological skills as well, since many clients are quite nervous, especially at first. This is a personal service that requires building a sense of trust with the client. You should be friendly, yet professional in demeanor.

There is a high demand for this service, and the opportunity to own your own business is quite good. There are not enough of us to meet the demand. That is always good news when looking for a career. Still, it takes two to five years to build a vigorous practice. It is possible to earn $150 to $200 an hour, but remember that you have business expenses to cover if you operate your own office.

When I meet new people, they are usually surprised to learn what I do for a living. During these discussions, I always focus on eye contact, since people tend to be self-conscious at first, particularly women. My guess is that they are concerned about their own situations. As a matter of fact, many do initiate more detailed discussions about my work, usually a little later and on a one-to-one basis.

What kind of marketing do you have in place to sell your business?

I have an ad in the yellow pages, and my business cards are available at several beauty salons and spas in the region. This location is quite central, so there is really no reason for a large sign outside, and it certainly doesn't say anything about hair removal. There is still a place for discretion, and clients who come in for the first time to discuss treatment or services seem to appreciate that.

A COSMETICS MANUFACTURER'S REP

My job title is Director of Salon Resources with a large East Coast supplier of beauty industry products. Let me say right away that this is a multimillion-dollar business with international clients, and I have a position of responsibility and respect that I would never have dreamed possible without college. I guess it just proves there are other ways to be a success in this business.

I started as a cosmetologist at the ripe old age of 20, and began to specialize in skin care and makeup. Within a year, I was working as an esthetician in a leading Florida resort area, while taking classes to get the salon owner's certificate. I worked hard and lived at home with my parents, saving every penny I could for my goal. It was a pretty spartan existence, but I knew what I wanted. At a time when lots of people my age are getting their first car loan, I had qualified for a $40,000 business loan and opened my own salon/day spa, also in a winter resort area.

I had always enjoyed attending beauty trade shows, since they are a wonderful opportunity to learn about the newest products and their application. It also became a chance to meet platform artists and manufacturer's representatives. The questions I asked and the level of interest I showed must have convinced some of them that I was a serious student of the industry, and before too long, these professionals began to ask for my résumé.

I began to explore what it would be like to go from owning a salon to working for one of the big corporations, and it had a certain appeal. I really didn't care for the business management side of what I was doing at the time, meeting with accountants and supervising daily details. My first assignment was as a national guest artist, presenting programs that used my technical skills in demonstrating the products, plus marketing know-how, since I was actually selling to the audience.

Of course, the artistic talents a cosmetologist develops over the years are always in use. Now I am something of a business executive and teacher. I travel once or twice each month, and I also write a column for the corporate newsletter, answering technical questions from the salon owners and managers who make up our client list.

For example, salons are clearly focused on ways to expand their base of services. My company is looking at several approaches. Hair coloring services are growing dynamically, as are fashion nails, waxing, and services related to preventing or dealing with hair loss.

Cosmetologists depend on steady customers, and as a group, those baby boomers are growing older every year. What interests them is looking young and fit, and you can see those concerns in the list of services I just mentioned. Next week, at our corporate training center, I begin presenting a series of workshops on haircuts that emphasize a fuller look for hair that is thinning. Of course, we have hair-care products that help alleviate this process. It's a natural avenue for salons to explore. After all, hair is their business. Clients are worried about thinning hair, and this is an area in which salons can increase their level of service.

Other new trends? Well, there is the nonsurgical facelift and the introduction of salon Shiatsu, a form of ancient Oriental massage. This is part of promoting a sense of well-being in salon services. It's ideal for busy people. Because the massage is administered while the client is fully clothed, it doesn't require much time, and once they experience the relaxation level that results, many who keep a standing appointment for hair-care services make an appointment for a massage on the same visit.

I am also involved in a series of training videos the company is making. My task is to work with our major clients, to discover the topics that their staffs are both interested in and can benefit from. Not every cosmetologist has time to travel to shows and workshops, so our intent is to put together practical information and *demonstrations that one or two staff members can watch, then put to use in their own work.*

My days are varied, and I must look my best with a minimum of fuss and bother. My work is always interesting, and I am in touch with a variety of people. The travel sometimes includes places such as New York, London, or Paris. Although the schedule permits little time for sightseeing, it's always exciting to be in a fashion capital when the new styles are introduced.

I think I've come a long way for someone without a college degree, but none of it would have been possible if I hadn't earned my cosmetology license and made a few sacrifices when I was first starting out.

MASSAGE AND THE COSMETOLOGIST

All cosmetologists learn something about massage in their general training. This skillful touch is meant to loosen stiff muscles, relieve pain, and provide relaxation. In cosmetology, massage is limited to the hands and feet, arms, scalp, neck, and shoulders.

"As a manicurist, I use massage techniques on the hands, arms, feet, and ankles of my clients. The ability to provide relaxation and a sense of well-being is part of the manicure or pedicure service," explains Diane, who works full time at a neighborhood salon.

"Occasionally, our estheticians perform facial massage and work on tense neck or shoulder muscles. I attend a yoga class at the YWCA, and through that connection I have given several workshops on the subject of infant massage. I have an eight-month-old daughter who had severe colic until we started daily massage sessions.

"Massage as a kind of therapy has a long history in most cultures of the world. Scientific studies prove that touch has healing properties, and I have certainly seen tense, cranky babies calm down during their sessions.

"Some of my clients have aches and pains from arthritis or repetitive stress injuries," says Anne Marie. "They find a massage soothing, particularly after soaking in warm paraffin."

Job opportunities for a massage therapist exist in such related fields as sports massage, where the object is combatting exercise-related injury, and infant massage, now recognized as a way to strengthen the emotional bond between parent and child and as a means to relieve stress.

Depending on state and local regulations, massage techniques may include the use of the therapist's hands, but also heat, light, water, or vibrating devices.

Giving a massage is strenuous work. The therapist must use correct body mechanics to avoid fatigue and work-related injuries. A cosmetologist with a calm, patient disposition is well suited to massage therapy.

In addition to private practice in homes or offices, the work environment may be part of a salon or spa, gym or health club, resort or cruise ship. Many massage therapists work with doctors or chiropractors, and a growing number of physical therapists and physicians employ them as well.

Massage can be found in some surprising locations. A chair massage facility was recently opened at Pittsburgh International Airport, and similar services are offered at various resorts. Hence, it is not surprising that the American Massage Therapy Association has stated that the popularity of massage is on the rise and that there are many jobs available in this field. The number of schools teaching massage in an

AMTA-approved program has more than doubled in the last decade. For additional information, consult the cosmetology school in your area, or the American Massage Therapy Association, P.O. Box 1270, Kingsport, TN 37662.

MEET TWO SUPERSTARS

Hair-shaping is an art. It takes a lot of practice and must be mastered before a student of cosmetology can qualify for work in the better salons. Vidal Sassoon said it best, "I think what we have done is changed hairdressing into haircutting. We made women aware of their possibilities."

Sassoon, who reigned over a world empire in hair style and hair care for more than forty years, is generally credited with elevating the haircut to an art form. From his London headquarters, Sassoon mastered a design created from geometrics forms. Scissors, a straight razor, a brush, and a blow-dryer were the basic tools. Practice proved to be the secret ingredient.

Stylists flocked to Sassoon's workshops and clinics, learning to create hairstyles that accented the client's best features. Soon the swingy, geometric cuts that gave hair motion and bounce were on the covers of all the fashion magazines, gracing the runways of high fashion shows in New York, Paris, and Milan.

Talk about practice—Sassoon spent almost nine years perfecting the short, swingy hairstyle that has become his signature look. Wash and wear hair became the rage, ignited by the short, short cut Sassoon designed for actress Mia Farrow. Soon the international jet set had joined the ranks of London shop girls and the smart city set trooping to his salon. The rest is hairstyle history.

Now an American citizen living in Los Angeles, Sassoon owns a chain of salons that bear his name and markets dozens of leading hair-care products. Sassoon is also credited with bringing increased respectability to the cosmetology business. Sassoon was a pioneer in the hairstylist-as-beauty-consultant movement. Before his time, few stylists spent much time analyzing the clients' features or discussing with them ways to achieve a hairstyle that worked best with their lifestyle and made the most of their features. Sassoon was among the first to use a hand-held dryer to achieve more fluid hairstyles. Along the way, he also invented the modern blow-dryer.

The two elements Sassoon believes are critical to a good haircut are time and talent. He believes a good cut, even by an experienced stylist, takes at least thirty to forty-five minutes. Haircuts at salons bearing his name are priced between $49 and well over $100, but clients can count on getting a look that reflects the founder's styling philosophy, since everyone on the Vidal Sassoon Salon staff is trained in-house.

What Vidal Sassoon did for hairstyling starting in the 1960s, Kevyn Aucoin is doing for makeup today. The Louisiana-born Aucoin, makeup artist to the stars, is the author of two books on the magic of makeup, and often uses before-and-after photos to illustrate his work.

Aucoin has expressed his opinion that no one needs a makeover and that there are no strict rules on using cosmetics. Instead, he prefers to make suggestions on how individuals can make the most of their natural looks.

Today, Aucoin operates in a world of professionals— models, photographers, the best lighting, makeup products from international beauty firms. These are elements he first admired in the Hollywood movies that fascinated him as a child.

His book *Making Faces* contains step-by-step descriptions of the looks illustrated, plus advice on how to achieve specific makeup effects. His earlier title, *The Art of Makeup*, features celebrity makeovers. Details on both titles appear in the section of this book called "For Further Reading."

9

Enjoying a "Day of Beauty"

A full-service salon or spa offers a complete array of beauty services and is an excellent place to observe professional cosmetologists at work.

Originally, a spa was more like a vacation resort, where guests traveled to another country or state to enjoy a sort of health vacation with a focus on improving health and beauty. These trips usually lasted for a week or more. Now the trend is toward shorter stays, closer to home. In 1999 alone, hundreds of new day spas have been built as part of chain hotel lodgings across the United States. Day spas associated with beauty salons are springing up at an even greater rate. As you prepare for your career in the beauty industry, it is possible that you will consider employment in one of these new ventures.

For our imaginary tour, let's say you have scheduled the exclusive "day of beauty" program. Along with a lot to learn, you have a great deal of pampering in store for you.

We approach the spa, part of a resort hotel—famous for its golf, swimming, tennis, and health club facilities—at 9 AM and enter an attractive reception area. The walls are decorated in a lively jungle print. The use of indirect lighting creates the effect of sunshine filtering through a leafy canopy of banana leaves and exotic blossoms. The sound system provides a rain forest background with gentle bird calls and the splash of a waterfall. Already, you sense a feeling of relaxation.

A well-groomed receptionist rises from her desk as you approach and greets you by name, smiling as she approaches to shake hands. You notice that her hair is shiny and lustrous, pulled back in a smooth chignon, and the hand that reaches out to you is smooth and soft, the manicure exquisite. After a brief confirmation of the services you have scheduled, the receptionist invites you to sample herbal teas or fresh fruit juice. In a matter of minutes, the esthetician, Lynn, with whom you have your first appointment, arrives, introduces herself, and escorts you to a small treatment room.

Lynn drapes you with soft cloth that will protect your clothing. She dons a white lab coat while she explains the steps you will undergo in her care. Her voice is soothing, her manner professional, as she describes the art of facial massage and exfoliation, a method of cleansing the pores in your skin. Your neck and shoulders relax under her practiced massage. Next she applies a heated botanical mask derived from seaweed, a sought-after treatment in the great spas of Europe. The green material is packed in an antiseptic-looking white glass container, with only a faint aroma of the ocean. Processed into a smooth, thick mass, it feels light as Lynn applies a generous coating to your chin, cheeks, nose, and forehead.

Lynn will be seeing another client during the twenty minutes you are undergoing facial treatment, but before leaving, she introduces Michelle, who will perform your manicure and pedicure. You have never before had a pedicure, and the gentle manipulation of

99

the reflexology massage is comforting. You have decided to have a silk wrap done on your fingernails, and Michelle moves on to this work with practiced ease.

Lynn returns, meticulously washes her hands, and applies to your eyes cotton pads that have been soaked in a cooling solution extracted from fresh cucumbers. She explains that this treatment is good for the delicate facial area below the eyes. Ten minutes later, you are still relaxing in the leather reclining chair when Lynn removes the eyepads. You feel noticeably refreshed, and it is time for you to choose just the right attractive shade of nail lacquer for your dramatic new nail length. Michelle offers some instruction on how to protect the artificial nails, and Lynn counsels you on the splash and pat approach to cleansing your face, morning and night. You are getting a clearer understanding of the role communication plays in being a professional cosmetologist.

Thus far, your face, hands, feet, and lower arms have been massaged and beautified. With your face newly cleansed, you are ready to move on to the hairstylist. When booking your appointment, you requested hairshaping and a body wave, using one of the new gentle formula waving treatments.

Lynn accompanies you to the hair salon, where you see a familiar face. Bryan, who cut your hair for two years while on the staff of a mall salon near your home, has recently been named manager of the styling center at this spa, and he is one of the reasons you scheduled this visit. Bryan's skill with a razor cut has given you the best-performing hairdo you've known in years, and you are willing to drive an extra fifteen minutes to stay in touch with such a talented hairstylist.

You have become part of Bryan's clientele, or following, a term used among cosmetologists to describe clients who are so loyal that they literally follow a favorite stylist, even when the pro changes jobs. The fact that Bryan has attracted a number of his former clients to his new job makes him a valuable asset to the spa staff. For example, you used to book just a wash and set at his former location, but now you are receiving more comprehensive services at the spa.

After a few minutes spent catching up and Bryan's assuring you that he loves this new assignment, you begin to discuss the hairstyle you are looking for and what you hope the body wave will do for the texture of your hair. Bryan shows you some photos from a styling guide, pointing out that he learned the technique from a platform artist at a recent, glamorous trade show in Houston. "That's the look for me," you agree. His enthusiasm makes you feel good about the change you are about to undertake, and you are confident in his ability.

You settle in for the shampoo and cut. Bryan has been trained in the Pivot Point method of cutting hair, and as you watch his reflection in the mirror, you notice that he repeatedly lifts sections of your hair with quick motions, comparing the left side with the right for balance and symmetry. Once your hair is cut and shaped, it is time to begin sectioning it for placement of the perm rods.

You notice that this new perm takes less time and has none of the smelly lotion associated with perms you've had in the past. When the processing is completed, you are back in the styling chair, where Bryan demonstrates how you can use the blow-dryer and a large round brush to achieve the same styling effects on your own.

One of the reasons you followed Bryan to his new location was the way he understands your hair-care needs, explaining in clear detail how to style your hair at home.

A year ago, Bryan introduced you to a new setting gel to tame the natural curl in your hair, and the results have been so great that you've been using it ever since. This is yet another reason you have such confidence in your stylist's ability.

Handing you a mirror, Bryan slowly rotates the chair to give you a look at your new hairdo from every angle. Perfect! And now it's time for a lunch break before your afternoon sessions.

The spa has its own dining room, with an atrium design. A fountain at its center is surrounded by flowering potted plants, and the menu features spa cuisine with healthy and freshly prepared offerings. You choose a salad course, and a mineral water as a beverage, followed by raspberry sorbet. There is plenty of time to relax before your next appointment, and no reason to be self-conscious because you are wearing no makeup—only salon personnel and other patrons are present in the private dining room.

Promptly at 2 PM, you return to the reception area and are shown to the makeup studio, where you are greeted by Julie, identified as a cosmetics consultant on the staff directory. Because you have always favored a conservative look, you pay particular attention to the way Julie has done her own makeup. It is reassuring to note the light, natural effect she has achieved. First, you learn about the color wheel, a palette of makeup shades ranging from pale to vibrant hues in a complementary, circular array. Julie demonstrates which tones best suit you. Next, Julie listens intently as you answer a series of questions about your lifestyle, time schedule, regular beauty routine, and whether you have ever had an allergic reaction to any makeup product.

You sit patiently while Julie expertly creates more of an arch in your eyebrows. This subtle change has given you a more alert, sophisticated look, you decide, admiring the results in the mirror. As the hour slips by, you are an intent student, learning how to handle a lip brush and blending color expertly on your cheeks. You agree to a slight change in foundation color, and you choose two new shades in lipstick. Julie has also taught you a new trick with eyeliner, taking full advantage of your newly enhanced brow line.

During the last ten minutes of your session, you learn how a few simple additions to your daytime makeup routine can transform it into a glamorous evening look. Then Julie explains how to take good care of your cosmetics. "They're an investment," she explains, packing your new purchases into a tiny gold-on-gold striped carrying bag bearing the spa's name in a bold script.

Your next stop is at the photographer's studio, where your fresh new look is captured in a series of glamour shots. You have brought along a change of clothes just for this occasion, and the session takes about an hour. The photos will serve as a reminder of this special day of beauty, in addition to guiding your hand as you replicate the hairstyle and makeup technique on your own.

The spa offers a buffet menu of services, and it had been difficult for you to decide between a Shiatsu massage or an aromatherapy session. Finally, you had decided on the latter.

It is late afternoon, and you start your first meeting with the aromatherapist. You learn that the inviting scents captured in tiny, jewel-like bottles are called "essential oils," which are derived from botanicals, or living plants. Some are exotic, found in abundance only in remote equatorial regions. Others may grow wild in meadows and home flower gardens.

Jennifer, a licensed cosmetologist who now specializes in this emerging field, explains that you have already experienced an aromatherapy treatment during your morning pedicure. "The lotion used in your foot massage contains essence of peppermint. Perhaps you noticed the aroma?" she asks. Thinking back, you do recall the pleasant tingling sensation and the invigorating aroma.

As the session goes on, you sample various oils made from plant parts such as petals, roots, leaves, and stamens. Some of the scents are familiar to you, others mysterious. You decide immediately that you like frangipani, sandalwood, and vanilla bean. A few drops in a hot bath or simmered in a potpourri, even in a candle—the drifting scents relax and soothe you.

Jennifer has increased her knowledge of aromatherapy by attending clinics and seminars, the most recent one in Paris, and her enthusiasm is contagious. She offers you an illustrated booklet on the subject, and you are pleased to accept it.

Before leaving the spa, you have one last appointment, with Jolie, a senior designer in the hairstyling salon who is also an expert in the art of body painting called Mehndi. Don't worry, you are not getting a tattoo; Mehndi is an ancient ceremonial art used in many cultures from ancient times, but originating in India, where it is still commonly used.

You greet Jolie and start asking the many questions you have about her art form. You know that the paste that is painted onto the skin is made from henna. "The paste we use is dried henna powder mixed with eucalyptus, clove, and essential oils," Jolie explains. Henna has been used safely for more than 5,000 years, she assures you, and the designs she creates last about a month, depending on how often the design is washed and the intensity of the original color application. The designs are derived from various ethnic cultures, including East Indian, Arabic, African, and Celtic peoples. These intricate painted symbols represent good health, fertility, wisdom, and spiritual enlightenment.

Jolie has a design portfolio that illustrates several examples. As you turn the pages, you see old-fashioned lacy bead choker necklaces, grapevines entwining an ankle, a chain of Celtic crosses encircling a bicep, hands painted to resemble lace gloves—palm and back—with nail polish to match.

"This is a folk art that is very old, yet here in the United States, it is very new as a form of adornment. It started on the West Coast, Los Angeles, mainly. If you were looking closely at the Academy Awards telecast, there were several celebrities with Mehndi body art to match their gowns," Jolie says.

"It doesn't require a license or official training, and with the new stencil kits, there's not even much artistic talent required. Just a steady hand and clients who are willing to try the technique. It's a perfect complement to high-fashion hairstyling or manicures, and because it is temporary, it doesn't require the commitment of a permanent design. I think it's fun, really."

After a look at the materials Jolie uses to create this art, you admit that one day you may want to try a design—just a small one though—and thank her for her time.

Leaving the spa, you pass a mirrored wall and pause a moment to fully appreciate your appearance. Your skin has a noticeable glow, your new hairstyle is vibrant and moves in a graceful line as you turn your head. Your hands are smooth and glamorous with the addition of long, newly lacquered nails. There is no tension in your neck or shoulders, and the spa cuisine you had for lunch was light, yet energizing. In addition to all this outward improvement, you have learned some quick and interesting methods on how to maintain your fresh new look. In addition, you have several new interests— botanicals, spa cuisine, and aromatherapy. While you came here to discover the secrets of a spa's day of beauty program, you are leaving with a renewed interest in cosmetology as a career. What you have seen and experienced has convinced you that being part of the beauty industry is the life you want to lead.

10

Toward a Global License

What does the future hold for cosmetologists? Leaders in the industry are working toward the day when graduates of cosmetology schools anywhere in the United States will meet the same set of educational standards, earning a license that will be recognized in all fifty states. Such a move is already under way in Europe, where professional cosmetologists will be able to cross international borders in pursuit of career goals.

Another factor in improving the beauty industry involves making it easier for new cosmetologists to get established in their profession. A recent survey indicated that most salons invest about $12,000 in training an entry-level cosmetologist in the first year of work. If the new employee had most of this training right from the start, salons could improve starting salaries instead, encouraging more of the promising cosmetology graduates to stay in the profession, achieve career goals faster, and help the salons that employ them thrive.

In recent years, several national beauty organizations, as well as educators, have come to the realization that good communication skills and an understanding of marketing are keys to success for entry-level cosmetologists. To ensure that adequate time is devoted to these topics during beauty school, a new National Skill Standard has been adopted across the nation. Cosmetology is the first area of career education to adopt a list of competencies for all of its students to master. As you read, keep in mind that this plan is designed to promote the image, growth, and development of professional cosmetologists.

FIVE CRUCIAL AREAS

Performance guidelines, divided into five critical job functions, are provided for the entry-level cosmetologist. They reflect not only the training you received in cosmetology school, but also what is expected of you on the job. The five areas are:

- Client service
- Business operations
- Product knowledge, use, and safety
- Fashion, art, and technical design
- Personal development

TWENTY PERFORMANCE GUIDELINES

These broad areas are further divided into twenty performance guidelines for entry-level cosmetologists. The following is reprinted with the permission of the Cosmetology Advancement Foundation:

1. Consult with clients to determine their needs and preferences as they relate to cosmetology services.
2. Conduct services in a safe environment and take measures to prevent the spread of infectious and contagious disease.

3. Interact with coworkers effectively and work as part of a team.

4. Manage time effectively in order to provide efficient client service.

5. Take necessary steps in order to develop and retain clients.

6. Market professional salon products effectively.

7. Maintain business records on client development, income, and expenses.

8. Use a variety of salon products safely while providing client services.

9. Manage product supplies efficiently for salon use and retail sales.

10. Provide basic manicure and pedicure services.

11. Provide basic skin-care services.

12. Apply cosmetics appropriately to enhance a client's appearance.

13. Provide a haircut in accordance with a client's needs or expectations.

14. Provide styling and finishing techniques to complete a hairstyle to the satisfaction of the client.

15. Conduct a color service in accordance with a client's needs or expectations.

16. Perform hair relaxation and wave formation techniques in accordance with the manufacturer's directions.

17. Provide nonsurgical hair additions.

18. Perform hair removal services.

19. Participate in lifelong learning to stay current with trends, technology, and techniques pertaining to the cosmetology industry.

20. Use appropriate methods to insure personal health and well-being.

The world of beauty is an interesting field in which to work, offering opportunities to express your personal creativity while becoming a skilled specialist. It is also a career that offers flexibility in work schedules plus many opportunities for entrepreneurs. With efforts to standardize licensing from state to state, cosmetology is becoming a truly portable career. Each day on the job offers the chance to improve a client's appearance, thus increasing that person's self-esteem. Seeing first-hand that one's own work is appreciated gives a boost to the cosmetologist's self-esteem, too.

Glossary

alopecia The deficiency of hair; baldness.

apprentice A person learning a skill or trade from an expert by working with that expert for a certain length of time.

aromatherapy Beauty treatments derived from fragrant botanical (plant) materials.

blending The physical act of fusing the color of hair during tinting and lightening applications.

chemical hair relaxer A chemical agent employed to straighten over-curly hair.

chignon A knot or coil of hair worn at the crown or nape, created from natural hair or a hair extension.

commission The percentage of money earned on sales that is kept by the cosmetologist.

competencies A determination of whether one's training meets a required level of accomplishment.

cosmetology The art and science of improving the hair, nails, skin, and products related to their care.

croquignole Winding of the hair under from ends to the scalp.

Egyptian henna A pure vegetable hair dye.

esthetician A cosmetologist who specializes in skin care and makeup arts.

fall An artificial section of hair running across the back of the head.

finger waving A method of shaping wet hair using only the fingers and allowing it to dry in place.

following A group of clients who are loyal to a certain cosmetologist because they like and trust him or her.

franchise A chain of salons with the same name and style of service, but individually owned.

generalists Cosmetologists who practice many or all of the various aspects of their training.

hair analysis An examination to determine the condition of the hair prior to a hair treatment.

hair texture The general quality of hair as to coarse, medium, or fine; the feel of the hair.

histology The study of animal and plant tissues.

internship Work experience while you study.

manicure The artful care of hands and nails.

marcel waving A method of shaping wet hair with clips and allowing it to dry in place.

massage Manipulation of the body by rubbing, pinching, kneading, tapping, to increase metabolism, promote absorption, and relieve pain.

master designer The highest level of designer in a salon.

nape The back of the neck.

pack A special cosmetic formula used to beautify the face.

pedicure Care of feet and toenails.

pigment Any organic coloring matter, as that of the hair, skin, iris.

pivot (hair-shaping) The exact point from which the hair is directed in forming a curve or shaping the hairstyle.

reciprocity A mutual agreement to exchange favors;

in cosmetology, it refers to different states accepting a cosmetology license issued in another state.

registered barber A person who has been trained in a certificate program for barbers.

résumé A written summary of a person's education, training, and work experience.

shaped haircut A haircut that uses layers to create a geometric shape.

shingling Cutting the hair closer to the nape of the neck and gradually longer toward the crown.

specialist Someone who concentrates on only one or two areas of cosmetology.

spiral winding Winding the hair from the scalp to the ends.

trichology The science of the care of the hair.

wrapping Winding hair on rollers or rods in order to form curls.

For More Information

American Association of Cosmetology Schools
901 North Washington Steet. Suite 206
Alexandria, VA 22314
(703) 683-1700
fax: (703) 683-2376
web site: http://www.thomson.com/aacs

American Massage Therapy Association
P.O. Box 1270
Kingsport, TN 37662
web site: http://www.amtamassage.org

Beauty and Barber Supply Institute
11811 North. Tatum Boulevard, Suite 1085
Phoenix, AZ 85028-1625
(602) 404-1800
fax: (602) 404-8900
web site: http://www.bbsi.org

Cosmetology Advancement Foundation
208 East 51st Street
New York, NY 10022

Joe Blasco Makeup Center
1670 Hillhurst Avenue #202
Hollywood, CA 90027
(323) 671-1085
web site: http://www.joeblasco.com

Future Cosmetologists of Houston Association
Ventura Ramirez, Advisor
HCCS Central College
1300 Holman, SJAC 115
Houston, TX 77004
(713) 718-6145
fax: (713) 718-6039
web site: http://www.ccollege.hccs.cc.tx.us

Los Angeles School of Makeup Designory
10153 Riverside Drive
Toluca Lake, CA 91602
web site: http://www.makeupschool.com

National Accrediting Commission of Cosmetology Arts
    and Sciences (NACCAS)
Arlington, VA
web site: http://www.naccas.org.

National Beauty Career Center
3839 White Plains Road
New York, NY 19467
(718) 330-1280

National Hairdressers and Cosmetologists Association
3510 Olive Street
St. Louis, MO 63103
(314) 534-1170

Spa/Salon Staffing
web site: http://www.beautytech.com.

The Studio Makeup Academy
1438 North Gower Box 14
Studio 308
Hollywood, CA 90028
e-mail: studiomakeup@earthlink.net

For Further Reading

Aucoin, Kevyn. *Making Faces.* New York: Little, Brown and Co., 1997.

———. *The Art of Makeup.* New York: HarperCollins, 1996.

Cotter, Louise; Dubose, Frances London. *The Transition: How to Become a Salon Professional.* Albany, NY: Milady Publishing Co., 1996.

Gately, Linda Athey, ed. *Salon Ovation's Cosmetology Dictionary.* Albany, NY: Milady Publishing Co., 1995.

Gearhart, Susan Wood. *Opportunities in Beauty Culture Careers.* Chicago: VGM Career Horizons, 1991.

Harper, Victoria. *Professional by Choice: Milady's Career Development Guide.* Albany, NY: Milady Publishing Co., 1994.

Hayden, Thomas, and Williams, James. *Milady's Black Cosmetology.* Albany, NY: Milady Publishing Co., 1991.

Lamb, Catherine. *Milady's Life Management Skills for Cosmetology, Barber-Styling and Nail Technology.* Albany, NY: Milady Publishing Co., 1996.

Lees, Mark. *Milady's Skin Care Reference Guide.* Albany, NY: Milady Publishing Co., 1993.

Milady's Standard Textbook of Cosmetology. Albany, NY: Milady Publishing Co., 1994.

Murphy-Martin, Mary. *Planning Your Cosmetology Career.* Englewood Cliffs, NJ: Prentice-Hall, 1993.

Rooks, Noliwe M. *Hair Raising: Beauty, Culture and African American Women.* New Brunswick, NJ: Rutgers University Press, 1996.

Rudman, Jack. *Cosmetologist.* New York: National Learning Corp., 1991.

———. *Rudman's Questions and Answers on the Occupational Competency Exam in Cosmetology.* New York: National Learning Corp., 1992.

Strazzabosco, Jeanne M. *Choosing a Career in Cosmetology.* New York: Rosen Publishing Group, 1997.

Wright, Crystal A. *The Hair, Makeup & Styling Career Guide.* New York: Samuel French, 1997.

Index